The Gene Guillotine

Kate Preskenis

The Gene Guillotine

AN EARLY-ONSET ALZHEIMER'S MEMOIR

✳

Kate Preskenis

PRESENT ESSENCE PUBLISHING

The Gene Guillotine: An Early-Onset Alzheimer's Memoir

Copyright © KatePreskenis, 2012

First published in the United States of America by Present Essence
Publishing

ISBN 978-0-9832948-0-1

Requests for permission should be addressed to:

Present Essence Publishing
info@KatePreskenis.com
www.KatePreskenis.com

Cover photo of Kate Preskenis is generous donation of a film
production company

Cover and Interior design by Joel Friedlander,
www.TheBookDesigner.com

Printed in the United States of America

DEDICATION

Dedicated to those who endure scientific research in hopes to end Alzheimer's disease; to those who give generously of their time, talent, and money to raise awareness, funds, and hope for fighting Alzheimer's disease; to caregivers who give endlessly; to executors of living wills who advocate for final wishes; to researchers working for a treatment and a cure.

~ In memory of Dick Preskenis and Maureen "Mo" Noonan Preskenis ~

TABLE OF CONTENTS

✳

✳

I Don't Know My Status

THE RESULT OF MY genetic testing for Alzheimer's disease sits at the National Institutes of Health (NIH). I can find out, or continue to wonder, trying to prepare. Somehow the dance feels safer. It is familiar; I have been on this merry-go-round year after year, revisiting what I have already seen. It is a haunting tone, but I am getting used to its eerie feel. Occasionally, I uncover new wisdom as my path gouges into the dirt; however, none of the pieces gathered have changed my life in a drastic way. Yet I still feel ill-prepared to go into the center fire.

This disclosure may not seem like much, but it has taken me years of writing, emotional wrestling, and numerous imagined pen names to reach this stage. Even now, I want to pull the book before it reaches reviewers, the book designer, the printer, you.

Through this book, I have chosen to reveal that my genetic status is unknown. By making my current situation public, I'm trying to reach out to other people with genetic diseases and to help educate about the emotional impact of early-onset Alzheimer's disease, also known as young-onset Alzheimer's disease. Do not ask anyone his or her genetic status. *Please read the Genetic Etiquette section of this book.*

I live under my own magnifying glass—a constant examination of my memory, choice of words, and emotional state. All aspects of my life are stifled by the knowledge that Alzheimer's disease in our family is linked to a specific traceable gene. Aptly called early-onset Alzheimer's, it begins to noticeably affect individuals in our family between the ages of 38 and 48.

Not knowing my status, I have chosen against committing to marriage, a career, or having children. Either I have it or I don't. The only thing I can change is my knowledge. Turning inward I look for strength required to know or not know. It is elusive and meanwhile, my life is waiting.

I've realized I had to write this book without knowing my genetic status. If I knew I had the gene, I wouldn't have had the courage or confidence to write; I would doubt my use of language, my judgment, my memory. If I knew I didn't have the gene, I wouldn't feel justified attempting to portray an accurate firsthand account, even in the past tense, if it no longer pertained directly to me. And I believe it is extremely difficult, if not impossible, to remember what it is like living with an unknown status once the knowledge is gained.

Within a month of Mom's death, I started writing this book—although at the time I had no idea it would actually be a book and didn't dare call it a book. I wrote because I didn't want to forget anything and I had this huge resource of journals and audio tapes.

When I began, I had just endured four months of life-changing events: my mom died of Alzheimer's disease, researchers at NIH found the genetic link to Alzheimer's in our family, and I survived my first round of Alzheimer's research including cognitive testing, blood draws, an MRI, and spinal tap.

I had thought my life would go back to normal after Mom died.

But, I felt so alone. My friends didn't understand losing parents at such a young age, much less the concept of genetic disease. I connected best with people over the age of 70. The only comfort I took was in Nancy Wexler's case studies of people affected by Huntington's disease. My siblings talked about Alzheimer's occassionally, but I thought of it constantly. I didn't want to bring up my fears, stirring up their own, if it was not already on their minds.

Writing became a therapeutic way for me to flush out my feelings. Plunking away on my brother's computer, I created a single-spaced 40-plus-page document. After establishing my commitment, I purchased my own computer with my share of Dad's life insurance money.

I've been in hiding for years, hiding so deep that in my recent eight-year relationship, I never disclosed all the details of my genetic heritage to his family or friends. If I didn't tell anyone in my new location, ignoring this disease, maybe my life would seem normal.

However, if I want the legitimacy of a memoir, I have to use my real name. If I want to connect with others, I have to be willing to be seen. A pen name would keep me safe but isolated; the trade-off is that I am tender, vulnerable, scared, exposed.

Last week, I was agonizing about possible negative ramifications of this book being out in the world. A sibling pointed out that I wasn't also recognizing the benefits. Maybe if we are lucky, this book will raise awareness of early-onset Alzheimer's disease, encouraging funding for research, which we can only hope will bring a cure for Alzheimer's.

If there is one thing I can give the world that no one else can, it is writing this book. I've written it from my memory and notes, my emotions, my perspectives at the time. I treaded carefully and meant no harm. It would be fascinating for each person in this book to write from his or her own unique vantage point. With all of my imperfection, faults, mistakes, strength, and passion, I hope you will hear my heart.

I Have Tried With All My Might to Tell You the Truth

My soul somersaults, leaving behind my grounded sentence.
Flip, flop, more to see, more to do.
More to write, but the writing is serious.
Too serious, in fact, to be read.
It will consume the naked heart with sorrow.
Watch your back, sadness creeps up.
It is all I have inside, yet my shaking knees may hide it forever.
I have tried with all my might to tell you the truth.
My heart would rather a kinder focus,
Twirling dances and passionate love affairs.
But my heart's stabbed wound bleeds.

Kate Preskenis
April 2012
Southern Oregon, USA

AUTHOR'S NOTE

✳

IN THIS BOOK, MANY names have been changed, including the names of doctors, nurses, researchers, caregivers, counselors, hospice employees, care facilities, and a hospital.

Names omitted:

I describe many private meetings between my siblings, our significant others, and extended family. Omitting the names and descriptive features of who said what in those chapters is to protect all of us while covering these important and delicate dialogues. The controversial issues contained within are politically sensitive, emotionally charged, and often fuel moral and religious debates. This applies to Chapters 22, 30, 33, 34, 35, and 36.

Sibling recollection:

Most of the book is told from my point of view. However, there are four chapters or sections of chapters that I have included in which I am not present. These chapters are important turning points in Mom's progression with Alzheimer's. This refers to Chapters 15, 17, 21, and 31. My siblings recalled various incidents that I captured on an audio recording. Later I transcribed these stories into chapter form and verified my written version with the siblings.

Researcher transcription:

Chapter 30, "Greedy Genes," is transcribed from video re-cordings. It is heavy in scientific research. This is presented to the reader the way I heard and experienced this life-changing news. Minor modifications to the dialogue have been made to ease un-derstanding in the written form.

Honoring the Significance and Privacy of Personal Genetic Information

RECENT ADVANCES IN TECHNOLOGY enable people to find out their genetic status of inherited diseases. Often, genetic information profoundly impacts an individual's life choices and his or her way of being in the world. It is an extremely intimate issue.

Unless you share your most private thoughts and feelings with each other, it is prying and inappropriate to ask about genetic status. There may be other ways to let a person know you care and want to support them.

If the individual chooses to share this with you, there may be a certain time and place for such a personal conversation. It is an honor to be trusted with such intimate information and you should be prepared and committed to keep the information a complete secret.

These tips may help you be supportive and sensitive to those who may or may not know their genetic status.

CHAPTER 1

✳

Family Legacy

BARREN MAPLE TREES AWAITING the first snowfall reach into the bleak gray sky. Their fallen leaves raked and bagged into black plastic slump against the foundation of our home, providing insulation for the coming winter. Our two-story white house is on Main Street. At the bottom of the hill, near the fire department, is the only stoplight in Adams. A block south is the ambulance squad and across the street is Belloff's Department Store, which opened in 1907 and now slopes and teeters over the creek. West of the light is the three-story Hotel Adams, the railroad tracks, and the Great Lakes Cheese manufacturing plant.

Beyond the train tracks is Interstate 81, our portal to the rest of the world. An hour south is Syracuse, and it is seven hours to New York City. Lake Ontario is twenty minutes west, accounting for the large accumulation of lake-effect snow that Adams receives each winter.

Dad, Mom, Dan, and I moved here two years ago for Dad's work and the exceptional public school system. My oldest brother, Bob, currently lives in Cape Cod and is actually my uncle. He is Mom's much younger brother and was still very young when his mom, my grandmother, became sick with Alzheimer's disease.

Later he was adopted into our family, taking the last name of Preskenis rather than Noonan. My sister Karen is nine years older than me and acted as a mini-mother, taking care of my emotional and physical needs; she lives and works in Pennsylvania near Aunt Fran, Mom's sister. My brother Jay is seven years older than me; he is in college. For holidays he organizes family football games and encourages our family to decide on movies by consensus. Todd is my new foster brother who has just joined our family and is three years older than me. Always joking and laughing, he threatens to plunge my head in the toilet when I get into senior high. I don't think he will, but still I'm scared he might. Dan is two years older than me and towers over me. Frequent moves to new schools have solidified our friendship as we stick up for each other and eat lunch together.

Six months ago when Mom and Dad showed Dan and me this rundown house, I held my nose. The smell started in the kitchen (sour milk and grease), continued in the bathroom (sewage), the attic (dust and rodents), and became worse in the living room (cat pee, wet dog, trash, and cigarette smoke). Old bubble gum was stuck to the floor. The furnace grate for the cold air return was removed so trash could be thrown directly into the basement garbage heap. This was the dirtiest place I had ever visited and there was no way I would ever live here.

Mom and Dad bought it anyway. Mom spent months ripping off wallpaper, sanding the hardwood floors, removing the wall paneling, taking out the false ceilings, putting in a new bathroom, and adding more electrical outlets. Dan helped consistently and Dad assisted when he wasn't working. I stayed in our rental home watching forbidden, sinful, and sexy soap operas.

Within four months, Mom made the house livable.

Now, in our cheerfully painted living room, I'm sitting in the worn wooden rocking chair that I was rocked in as an infant when Dad used to sing, "Lula lula baby, lula lula Katie." I'm in eighth grade. Blonde hair, blue eyes, and fair-skinned, I'm easily recognized as Maureen's daughter. Braces line my teeth, a luxury on which Mom and Dad decided to splurge.

My mom, nicknamed Mo, is sitting behind me on the plaid polyester couch. Gentle smile lines cannot be hidden on her unusually solemn face. Wearing her standard attire, a turquoise rescue squad shirt and a pager clipped to faded men's Levi's, she is sitting on the edge of the couch, pressing the cushion flat against the pine wood frame. Her elbows are braced on her knees; her calloused fingers are clamped together while her thumbs chase each other in tight circles. She is perched like an athlete waiting for the pep talk before the big game.

In the darkened living room with the shades drawn tight, the movie begins. It is a worn recording and the color is mostly brown and off-white, sort of like a black-and-white that's trying to be color but doesn't quite make it. The fuzzy sound forces me to sit within four feet of the TV speaker to make sense of the garbled words. The picture flashes up and down. Playing with the tracking button to no avail, I strain to see the jumpy images on the monitor. My heart pounds in my chest and goose bumps rise on my arms. My mind is as erratic as the picture, wondering what is about to take place.

It is a movie anyone would give up on and say isn't worth watching. However, there was intensity in Mom's voice that I have never noticed before when she somberly requested, "Katie, I need you to watch *Do You Remember Love?* starring Joanne Woodward. It's about Alzheimer's disease, the disease that took my mother before you had a chance to know her."

I watch the husband find things that his wife has put away in absurd places: the dustpan in the refrigerator and the iron in the freezer. Her cabinets are labeled "cups," "glasses," "plates," but it makes no difference; she still opens them anyway, searching for the right thing, which is soon forgotten when something more interesting catches her attention.

It is the gentle *whoooft* of a tissue coming out of the box that slides on the marred brown coffee table that brings me back into the room. Between scenes Mom blows her nose the way she taught me when I was younger, first one nostril and then the other before wiping underneath. I don't dare turn around. I have seen her cry only one other time.

Secretly, I'm thankful to be in front of Mom so she can't see my smirks at this absurd comedy. Trying not to think about Mom's crying, I watch the woman on the screen. She is walking through a park alone, weaving through people until fixating on a small pond of water. Suddenly, she takes off her jacket and runs to the pond as children step aside. Jumping up and down, she's laughing and intentionally splashing the nearby children and parents. She takes off her blouse, but doesn't pay attention to the fact her trousers and camisole are getting wet.

I am laughing out loud, but it's nervous laughter. This movie is crazy. Mom's crying. I don't know how to respond. This hilarious actress is childlike and playful in the uptight adult world. I love that she is clothed and splashing in the water. Purposefully trying to ignore the translation to my own mother doesn't work.

Is this how Grandma acted? I know she had Alzheimer's and forgot stuff, but she died when I was three. I never knew her or anyone else with Alzheimer's disease. Grandma Jean, my grandmother's best friend, became Grandpa Noonan's new wife and took her place in my mind. I didn't miss her. I didn't ask about her. I did know she liked the beach, singing, and being with her sisters. *Will Mom get this disease, and the unraveling of her life, personality, and relationships that go along with it?* My stomach tightens. I'm afraid to move and my breathing gets shallow.

In the next scene, the woman is whimpering and wrapped in

a blanket at the police station. The husband comes in with a bag of dry clothes and says, "It is me, George. Do you know who I am?"

She has a blank face. He continues, "I'm your husband."

She blinks her eyelids closed and looks away. "I know that."

"If you are going to do things like this, I'm going to have to take the car away from you."

The woman's lips form a thin line, the corners drawing down. Her nose flattens as she continues to whimper and murmur.

Later that same evening, the husband gets off the phone with the president of the university where his wife teaches. He sits down next to his wife and tells her, "They are going to let you go."

"Go where?" she asks.

"They are taking you off the teaching staff permanently."

"Because I was in the wet today?"

"Water, not wet," he corrects. Then he lowers his head. She consoles him.

When the credits come up, I sit still as a stone, scared to move, and wonder if I will see these traits in my own mother. I'm afraid to look at her, so I pretend to stare at the indiscernible names that flutter on the screen.

Mom breaks the silence. "Katie, do you have any questions?"

Quickly, I answer, "No."

Mom proceeds, "What do you think of the movie?"

Breathing in all the courage I can muster, I turn toward this woman, my mother. I burst into sobs. "Mom, you can't get this! I need you."

Reaching out a hand, Mom guides me next to her on the couch. Her rough hand strokes my face. "I'm well now. There is a chance I could get it, but they think it skips a generation, so I should be fine. I only wish you didn't have to worry about it."

I take a deep breath. Hearing that it skips a generation calms me; I don't care about me, at least not yet.

Mom continues, "Katie, we think it is passed down to children from the parents because both your grandma and her sister had it. They shared genes being identical twins."

I shudder, praying that Mom will stop talking about genetics. This movie and conversation is as awkward as our introduction to sexuality talk with Christian audio tapes. I don't know where she is leading.

"My mother lived for years in the fetal position after her brain function decreased. The hospital kept her alive with tube feeding and IVs."

"She lay in bed not doing anything?" I ask in disbelief. Mom never talks about Grandma.

"Yes, she didn't recognize her kids and couldn't talk or do anything. She was a vegetable."

I watch Mom's mouth move beneath her reddish nose, glistening eyes, and short white hair. Her hair, like this conversation, is a testament to her life: clean, organized, and practical. The words I hear, but I don't quite understand.

"Katie, I don't ever want to be kept alive like that. I want to be allowed to die. In fact, I would rather kill myself. If I can't eat on my own, I don't want to be fed. I don't want to live."

"Does Dad know you feel this way?" I ask, while also wondering if my siblings have seen this movie. Mom is never like this—emphatic, revved up, pointed, and teary.

Mom's reply is brash. "Of course, Dick and I have talked about this."

My voice shakes. "Mom, you're making me uncomfortable. Do you mean you want to just die?"

"Yes, Katie, if I have a terminal disease or end up in a vegetative state from an accident, I want to naturally die without medical intervention to prolong my life," she states, smacking her right fist like a judge's gravel on the coffee table. "Let. Me. Go."

CHAPTER 2

Lucky

ARRIVING HOME FROM INDOOR track practice my junior year of high school, I'm met by Dad in the kitchen. His black hair salted with gray is short and professional in the front; the back is pulled into a low, curly ponytail. His bearded round baby face takes ten years off his age.

"Katie, are you okay? Do you want to talk?" He searches my face and takes a step toward me, and as I hug him my eyes moisten. I can't escape his keen glance with my hastiness to get to my room and be alone. Like a sixth sense, he always knows when I'm upset.

"I'm fine," I say unconvincingly as I walk out of the room.

In the next room, Mom is sitting at the dining room table. It is draped with material, patterns, and pins. *Duddduda duddad duddda.* Mom's eyes dart sideways for a brief second, noticing me, and then immediately back to the stitching hum of the Singer machine.

"Katie, I need you to try this on before I go much further." Her body is bent forward and reading glasses perch on her nose. She is working beneath the tiny light of the needle arm.

"Okay," I say with the slightest smile. Mom's talent has already worked magic. "I'm sweaty," I tell her, meaning that I don't feel like trying on the dress.

"That's okay," Mom says, getting up from the table and following me to my room.

The silky rayon lining slips gently over my thighs and I wiggle slightly to get the narrow waist over my butt. The straps hug my shoulders. Touching the outside of the dress, it feels like the tender petals of a rose. I glance in the bedroom mirror at the burgundy velvet dress with a white satin shawl adorning my shoulders and covering my bust. I catch Mom's eye.

"I love it, Mom, it is so beautiful. It's almost done. You must have worked on it all day."

Mom zips it up and checks the seams. "It's beautiful on you. I'm glad you like it. Stand on this chair so I can get the hem line right."

Cautiously, I climb while yanking up the dress to allow movement. I feel like a princess, despite the white sweat dried on my skin. The shawl's cool, slippery satin makes me look like I have boobs. It comes together in the front so it pulls my chest in a bit and the satin flares out, making my bust appear at least a size bigger.

"Mom, thanks for making this for me! It's so nice not to have to borrow another dress, and try to find one that I like and fits me."

We are silent as Mom measures from the floor to the bottom of the material. Then she leans away to scan the length. Next, she examines the hem in detail and says, "Katie, it seems like you had a hard day."

Caught off-guard, I sigh heavily, remembering. "Yes. I don't know what to do. I'm struggling with guy stuff." I hesitate; we haven't talked much about guys, and lately when I tell her something, she forgets within a month.

"Hmmm," she says. "Turn to the right a bit." She waits, knowing I will talk when ready.

"I feel like I should get back together with a guy I was seeing." I don't want to tell her who. A couple of weeks ago, Mom said something in front of Dan and Todd about a guy I used to like. Dan already knew because I ask his advice. I'm sure Todd suspected my crush, but her comment was way too revealing for my comfort zone.

"Do you want to?" she asks with three pins between her teeth.

"I don't know; he is cute and nice. But it's also complicated because a close friend likes him too."

"That does make it difficult. Do you really like *him*, or is he merely someone to be with right now?"

"I feel content, but all my feelings are short-lived." Some days I really like him and other days I think he is fine as a friend.

"Turn the rest of the way around. Good, hold still." Mom scans the hemline one last time. "Good. I'll hem it, let the waist out a little, finish the zipper clasps, secure the stays, and then have you try it on again."

"Okay," I say while playing with the floppy white collar, "is there any way to boost it up a smidge?"

"Let me see." She flips the collar up, pushes it around, scrutinizes it in the mirror at the side angle, squishes it in, and finally says, "Oh, that will be easy as long as you are willing to keep this down. It won't look pretty if the flap flips up, but I can add a piece of bunched netting to give it some lift."

"I don't want it huge, I want it—"

"I know, you want it just right," she laughs.

"Yeah, just right." Mom makes do with whatever is on hand. I like to be prepared and have everything perfect.

Holding onto the velvet and satin Christmas ball dress, I delicately let my nearly bare body ease out of the pin-filled material. Mom reaches out to take it and squeezes my outstretched hand. Then, she leaves to work on the dress.

Mom knows what to say and what not to say to get me to open up, letting her in on my life. I put on my stinky track clothes to walk to the shower. *Duddda*, the sound of the sewing machine fast at work vibrates through the house.

A month later, I'm coming home from school and Mom is standing in the kitchen. The smell of homemade chicken soup and yeast hang in the air. "Hi Mom." Then, looking around for a minute I ask, "Where is Lucky?"

"A lady came today to get the dog," Mom states without emotion.

"Huh? Was it really her dog?" I ask. We have had the dog for two weeks after waiting the appropriate length of time to adopt it from the dog catcher.

"It appeared so; Lucky went to her when she called."

"But Ma, that dog will go to anyone. It's friendly."

Mom shrugs and continues to knead the bread for the four waiting pans.

I can't shake the feeling that Mom gave away our dog and doesn't seem to care. I have wanted a pet for years, but we couldn't afford one. The last pets we owned were chickens, pigs, barn cats, one cow, a horse, and a big, mean dog named Trevor. That was on the farm in Iowa and we left when I was two.

Mom doesn't seem ready to talk and I have nothing more to say. My hands clench; I move away.

An hour later, I hear Dad's Mitsubishi Galant backing into the driveway. I walk toward the kitchen, mostly so I can hear first-hand what he has to say about Mom giving away Lucky.

When Dad walks inside, Mom turns off the water, drying her

hands. Dad asks, "Hi Maureen. How was your day?"

"Hi Dick, it was good, how was yours?" They hug and peck on the lips.

"Fine. Thanks for asking."

Mom resumes washing the carrots and cabbage for coleslaw. I'm standing in the doorway between the kitchen and dining room. Dad hugs me and then peers toward the living room, naturally expecting Lucky to be nearby.

"Lucky, come here Lucky."

Wide-eyed, I stand silent. Ten seconds go by, but Lucky never comes to Dad's call. I want to tell him, but I'm waiting for Mom to talk.

"Where's Lucky?" Dad asks. Mom, busy with the food processor on the front of her KitchenAid, keeps working, dropping in the veggies, pushing them through, and catching them in the stainless steel bowl.

"Oh, a lady called today and claimed the dog," Mom yells over the grinding noise.

"What did she say?"

"She said she was the owner of the dog and would be by to get him later." Mom keeps changing the story. She told me that the woman simply stopped by the house, but didn't say she had called first.

"You let Lucky go? Did you call the dog catcher to verify her story?"

"Yeah, oh, I don't know. The lady came and it was obviously her dog—Lucky went right to her. What could I do?" Mom answers quickly and unplugs the mixer.

"Maureen, how come you didn't wait until we could say goodbye to Lucky? Do you have her number?"

"Uh, no, I don't think so, she claimed the dog." The details of Mom's day are becoming more and more simplified.

Dad's face grows tight and his lips press together. Steam pours off the soup as Mom removes the cover, quickly stirs, and then covers it again. We had gone through all the proper channels and waited long enough to adopt the apparent stray that had been roaming busy Main Street for days.

"Did she say why she left the dog and had not claimed it until now? How do you know Lucky will be taken care of and not abandoned again?" Dad is following Mom around the kitchen from the mixer to the stove to the sink. His voice is a notch above normal. Respect and mild temperament still dominate his words despite his frustration. He never yells, curses, or uses physical aggression. Dad's pointed assertive questions reveal he was getting attached to Lucky. I thought Dad was simply tolerating Lucky so I could have a dog.

Mom shifts nervously, thinking about the day. Then she says, "All I know is the woman showed up, Lucky went to her, and she took Lucky. It was her dog."

I'm angry, hurt, and confused. *Why is Mom being weird, distant, aloof, secretive, hiding all the important details? Her behavior is strange. Why does she keep baking, grinding, and cooking rather than stopping to talk with us when we are both obviously upset? What is she hiding? Did she not like the dog and tried to get rid of it?*

CHAPTER 3

✳

Highway to Devastation

A WICKER BASKET BALANCED between my hip and arm is bulging with dirty clothes. I'm doing laundry and packing for my first year of college. St. Lawrence University is a small liberal arts school located an hour and a half from home. I've picked this college for its generous scholarship, location, as well as familiarity, having attended a leadership conference and indoor track meets there. Even though it is small, I'm nervous I'll get lost amid the 500 freshman after graduating from a high school with only 120 students.

On my way to the washer and dryer, I walk past Mom in the bright blue kitchen that matches the color of her eyes and she asks, "What does your shirt say?" I pause, putting down the basket to properly show off the shirt. She reads it and has me turn around so she can read the back too. "'Highway to your dreams,'" she reads aloud. "Where did you get that?"

Proudly, I tell her, "Jim gave it to me; he was given it at Canisius College orientation last week before starting football camp." Jim and I are high school sweethearts. We started dating the end of our junior year. He is tall and handsome with short, curly blonde hair, sky blue eyes, and a fit muscular body that is tanned from lifeguarding this summer.

"It's cool," she says, a bit outdated in her hip lingo. I smile, feeling "cool" wearing my boyfriend's clothing, and scamper off down the wood steps, aware of how this t-shirt moves on my body. Barely noticing the damp basement smell, I try not to get any of the hanging cobwebs on me. I throw the clothes in the wash and run up to the second story of the house to sort through the photos I want to bring to college.

BEEEEE Deet, dee tat leet tat leet ... familiar tones ring through the house as Mom's pager sounds and she darts out to an ambulance call. Her car starts, and a second later she flies out of the driveway and down the hill. She is one of the many volunteers who keep the ambulance running in our small community.

Upon her return two hours later, I meet her in the kitchen, soaking in all the time I have left with her until I leave for St. Lawrence. We talk briefly about the motor vehicle accident and then to my dismay, she glances down at my shirt and says, "'Highway to your dreams'. That's cool, Kate. Where did you get that? Turn around so I can see the back."

I'm surprised, but I figure she is distracted from her call. I answer her, "Jim gave it to me; it's from his college orientation last week."

I turn ever so slowly, absorbed in thought, wondering if we are really repeating the same conversation. *Did she forget I was wearing this shirt earlier today? Is she noticing something new about this shirt?*

Normally at this point, she will begin to remember something as being familiar and ask if I have worn it before, but she says nothing. She raises her eyebrows with enthusiasm that I cannot return.

Curious, I say, "Was that call stressful?"

"Nah, the standard injuries—a sore neck, a couple of cuts, and a trip to the hospital."

Puzzled, I walk upstairs wondering why she hadn't listened to me tell her about this shirt earlier. Slowly sitting down on my bed, I notice the air is thick with dust from packing. My mind isn't on college, but on all these recent weird interactions with Mom.

An hour later, Mom hollers up to my room and asks if I will be home for dinner. I yell "Yes!" and suddenly realize my load of laundry is probably done. At the top of the cellar stairs, I open the door to the dimly lit spider haven as Mom is coming from the freezer with chicken for dinner.

A bit out of breath, she asks, "Is that a new shirt?" nodding to the one I am wearing.

I stare at her. I can barely speak, but manage to stammer, "I … it's from Jim's college." She asks me to turn around as she has two previous times today.

Eerily reading aloud, "'Highway to your dreams,'" her voice trails off as she seems to be thinking and taking in the information for the first time.

I'm stiff, and fear oozes into me as if from the cellar, slowly creeping up my legs and into my core. I don't say much. Gingerly, I walk down the stairs, scared and angry. Taking my fluffed, toasty laundry out of the dryer, I'm careful not to drop any on the dirt floor. The words "highway to your dreams" are repeating over and over in my mind in Mom's thoughtful tone. I clench my jaw and swallow so hard it hurts my throat. My body moves up the familiar stairwell without seeing, my eyelids are fixed open, and I have stopped breathing. I make it all the way to my room before drawing in the breath that becomes sobbing tears with the exhale. I drop the clean clothes on the floor.

Hands shaking, I rip off the shirt and change into an old familiar t-shirt that I have worn for years. Both fists clench around the innocent cotton material, wringing it to make it take back all I have just experienced. I throw the white, wadded-up shirt against the opposite wall. Stumbling over my clean clothes to find my pillow, I bury my face to squelch the screams that billow from my throat. The wailing stains my cheeks, and ever so slowly I reach to the shirt and clutch it to my chest.

The personality changes, the occasional memory loss, and confusing interactions can all be explained away. But today, I saw the sign I have been waiting for and at the same time hoped would never come. I want to know that I'm not going crazy, but also don't want my worst fear confirmed.

My 50-year-old mother has Alzheimer's disease.

✳

CHAPTER 4

Permanently Borrowed

TWO MONTHS LATER, DAD walks up the gray cement path to my freshman college dorm. I embrace him with a huge hug. He gives me the rose he is carrying.

"Dad, thanks so much!" I open the card. It reads, *Thinking of you. I am glad you are my daughter.*

Glowing, I pull out scissors and cut the stem. Then I ease the delicate red rose into a Nalgene bottle before placing it on my desk.

Pointing to a stack of papers, I say, "Dad, we have to write another letter to the financial aid department. They say that I'm your dependent because you claimed me on your taxes last year. They don't care that I'm paying for college by myself."

"Let's write the letter now, then go to dinner, and we will take it to them tomorrow." He pulls out the wooden desk chair and sits down to read the newest correspondence.

"Don't you have audits all day tomorrow?"

"That's okay, I will rearrange my schedule." Dad has intentionally asked for extra work in St. Lawrence County so he can spend time with me.

We spend the next hour on the letter. I miss Mom; it would

have taken her half the time, but Dad rereads all the past communication. She helped my oldest siblings with all their college paperwork, but is unable or unwilling to help with mine. Dad is disorganized compared to Mom, but I would rather him help me than have to do it all by myself.

Driving to the dorm after dinner, Dad softly says, "I miss you now that you are not at home."

"Thanks, I miss you too." Then the sincerity sinks in. He doesn't mean it in the way I always assumed, that he is my dad and has to love me. He gains as much from this relationship as I do. Intense joy zips through me with this new realization.

Before getting out of the car, I reluctantly give Dad his brightly colored plaid flannel shirt that I have borrowed for the past month. I felt guilty borrowing it, because he doesn't have many clothes. I like having something of Dad's to wear when I have a hard day, as a constant physical reminder of his love. When I put it on, I feel like I'm getting one of his warm hugs.

"You can have it Kate," he says, attempting to hand it back.

After thinking for a moment, I say, "No, I don't want to have it. I want to borrow it from you, if you don't mind."

Dad restates, "You can *have* it!"

Taking it from him, I say, "Thanks, but I would rather borrow it from you than own it myself. I wouldn't enjoy wearing it nearly as much if it didn't belong to you."

Finally understanding what I'm saying, Dad chuckles, "Well then, you can borrow it permanently."

Home from college for the weekend, I look out our dining room window and see daffodils blooming from the moist ground near the garage. The last of the snow has melted. Mom and I are hovering over the sewing machine for the second weekend in a row, making a prom dress.

My friend Gary, a senior in high school, has asked me to go with him. I miss high school where I was somebody: class president, in honor society, co-captain of varsity soccer, homecoming queen, and voted "most school-spirited."

Mom's busy moving her hands, adjusting the bright blue rayon in all directions. She stops suddenly and stares at me blankly.

"What was I going to do?"

Taking in a breath I say, "We are putting in the zipper." I wonder if it would be quicker if I did it myself, but I don't have the confidence or the skill that Mom has. I fold up the tissue paper pattern and return it to the envelope. I wish I could take the cutting edge from my voice. My lower gut aches.

Mom lets out an exasperated sigh. She snatches the thread ripper and removes her most recent stitching. I was excited to have her make me another dress, but watching her struggle is torture. Earlier today, Mom said she couldn't balance the checkbook. A deep, throbbing sadness lingers over my entire being. I hate the fact that Alzheimer's is a lurking presence, yet still a taboo dragon.

"Okay, I think we are ready," she says, holding the zipper. I cautiously inspect her work, trying to stay grateful that she is doing this for me. It has to be ready next week.

I undress quickly and slide the material over my shoulders.

"I'll zip it up for you."

"Thanks Mom. I love this color, it's my favorite."

Walking around me and surveying the dress, she inquires, "What's next?"

"We have to measure the spaghetti straps and begin to figure out the length."

Mom takes the straps from the table and hands me the pincushion. It's amazing she knows how to do all the individual pieces but when the whole dress is in front of her, she can't figure out which detail needs to be done next.

Once she finishes, I ask, "How are the sides, can we take them in a smidge?"

"We can do anything."

She grabs two more pins from the white crocheted pincushion in my hand, and pulls the dress up to reach the inside seams on my right side. Then she moves to the left side.

"How's that?"

"It feels better. This right strap feels looser than the left."

"We can't have that now, can we?" Mom says, pulling to re-adjust the pin.

"Mom, thanks for making this for me. I'm sorry I'm uptight, I just want it to come out right." I feel guilty wanting the dress perfect—Mom is doing her best. It is my only option. I can't afford to buy one. I know this is taxing Mom, especially with her faltering abilities. It is weird to see the changes in her just by comparing this dress to the velvet dress of two and a half years ago. I wonder if she notices the changes too. I feel mean, sad, and frustrated on the inside and am trying to be patient, tolerant, and loving on the outside. She isn't faltering on purpose; it is the disease, but it feels so personal because it affects my immediate life now.

"I know Kate, it will be fine."

I appreciate her optimism, but it doesn't convince me. "Hey, this front is weird. It gaps funny when I hunch forward."

"It sure does." Mom inspects it. "I have an idea. Let me pin the middle of the front."

"What's that for? What are you doing?"

She smirks. "You'll see. Give me the dress."

Reluctantly, I hand her the dress at arm's length, squinting in nervous anticipation. She takes out a single piece of thread and begins to hand sew down the center of the dress. She sews for about four inches. Then, pulling on the thread and pushing the material, she gathers it all together. I cringe, not wanting her to mess anything up. Boldly, she ties a knot in the thread.

"Okay, try it on again."

Apprehensively, I step into the dress. Instead of it being like a uni-boob sports bra, she has accentuated the chest by gathering the center. "Mom, it's great, but how can I be sure that single thread won't break when I'm dancing?"

"That's temporary; we can reinforce it. I wanted to be sure you liked it first."

"How did you think of that?" I ask, amazed.

"I dunno, some ideas just pop in my head. I don't know where they come from. Now, what are we doing next?"

✳

CHAPTER 5

Dr. Whitlock

MOM AND I ARE doing errands and I need a medical exam to be allowed to run cross country this fall in my sophomore year of college. Mom insists, "We will drop by the doctor's office to see if they can squeeze you in."

"Is that allowed? I feel like we're imposing if we don't call ahead."

"Ah, nonsense, they will tell us if they don't have space."

We take turns reading the *Reader's Digest* jokes to each other in the examination room. It is not unusual for us to pal around together, so I don't think anything of it. Our laughter echoes in the small room until we hear a file and clipboard clang against the door.

The tall, fast-talking doctor enters the room, his belt pulled around his big belly and his shirt tucked in tight. He is in his usual hurry.

He starts with small talk. "How have you been? Mo, are you on call this weekend?" His office assistant is also a volunteer on the ambulance squad. Then he jumps to why I am here. "So you need a physical?"

He follows the check-off list issued by my college and laughs.

"This is merely to see if you are breathing." He begins with my eyes. Getting right next to my cheek, I feel his heavy breath on my face. I always feel like he is going to try to kiss me and I'm totally grossed out. I can barely sit still. Then, before I flinch away, he continues to my ears and throat. Testing my reflexes, he bangs on my knees and even jokingly tests my elbow. My lungs are next with the icy cold stethoscope.

"Well, you're alive," he says, beginning to sign the college papers.

It is a carefree atmosphere, until out of the nowhere Mom urgently says to the doctor, "Tell her I don't have Alzheimer's disease."

The doctor's forehead furrows with confusion. He turns to Mom and then to me. My face is blazing hot; I had no idea Mom would talk about this in front of him. Sure, I had mentioned to Mom that I was concerned about the changes I was seeing in her, but I thought I hadn't talked about it much. I assumed that it was one of those subjects we only talk about at home, alone.

With the *Reader's Digest* scrolled tightly in her hands, Mom says, "She thinks I have Alzheimer's disease; tell her I don't have the disease."

I feel like a deer in the headlights, frozen, stalked. I wonder what he will say. *If he asks any questions,* I think, *I can't answer truthfully about the symptoms I see; I can't betray Mom like that in public. Her reputation at the ambulance squad is at stake. What is she doing?*

The doctor who had minutes before been busy moving equipment, giving his signature, shuffling papers, remains static as if there is a loaded gun to his head. There is an ironic physical peace in the mostly white room, despite the emotional and psychological chaos exploding inside each of us. Suddenly, I wonder if he sees the signs too, and is wondering how to break it to her.

That thought vanishes as his eyes narrow. He looks at me, taking hold of the loaded gun. Pulling the trigger with all his degreed authority, he emphatically states, "Your mother doesn't have Alzheimer's disease. You don't know what you are talking about."

I am wounded, unable to respond, bewildered, alone. The exam is over and the doctor bustles out the door. My body slides heavily off the exam table and my feet drag across the floor. My stomach churns as Mom, talkative and elated, signs a check for the co-pay. The doctor darts into another exam room. My spirit hovers over my body, wondering if it is safe to come back. The waiting room is packed but thankfully, I don't recognize anyone.

When I slide into the passenger seat of the red '82 Toyota, I want to look at Mom in the driver's seat, but I don't want to encourage conversation. With my peripheral vision, I can see her eyes through the angle of the rearview mirror. She is focusing on driving. I turn and look fully at her face. Smug, content, resolute, her expression indicates the conversation is over. My mind races. If what the doctor said is true, that my mom does not have Alzheimer's disease, then does Mom not care about me anymore? Is she intentionally being mean? What else could be wrong with her?

We never mention that interaction again and it will be months before I gain the courage to point out her forgetfulness.

CHAPTER 6

Forced Underground

GROGGY FROM SLEEP, I feel a warm hand on my shoulder.

"Kate, it's Dad," he whispers to not alarm me, but I already know it is him from his peaceful presence.

Waking to the weighted slant of my mattress from where he is sitting, I see his silhouette in the glow from the hallway. I smile. It is still dark outside, and I'm huddled under the heavy covers in my twin bed. The red light of the digital clock shows 4:00.

It is early January, a few weeks before I return to St. Lawrence for the last semester of my sophomore year. I attended Jefferson Community College the first semester of my sophomore year due to a back injury. I missed St. Lawrence, but loved attending the same college as Dan, eating lunch, studying in the library, and going to parties where he was called Wild Dan and I was Crazy Kate. Dan and I have been talking about Mom's symptoms for a couple of years. Only weeks have passed since Dad has finally recognized Mom's symptoms as Alzheimer's. Despite Dad's long denial, I have felt immense support and connection with Dan. However, Dan is moving to Oregon at the end of this year to finish school and I'm a bit panicked with him leaving. Then I'm the last one close to home, by myself.

"Hi, Dad," I mumble.

When I was in junior high, I hated waking up; I was a miserable grump. This is different. I'm grateful to be awakened, even after only four hours of sleep.

"I'm getting up to finish paperwork, Mom is asleep, and I'm wondering if you want to talk. Don't feel like you have to; I know you are tired, but you did ask me to wake you."

"Yeah, I do. I'll be down in a minute," I say, pointing my toes and reaching my arms overhead in a full body stretch.

Dad leaves and shuts the door. I turn on the lamp near my bed and pull on baggy navy sweatpants that Mom has patched twice. I grab a sweatshirt and a pair of socks. The air is chilly. I stumble slightly as I walk down the hall. It jolts me out of my sleepy stupor, and, realizing one creak from the floorboards may cause Mom to stir, I continue slowly down the slippery wooden stairs.

Mom is jealous of our time together; she doesn't like being left out and has a hard time being alone. We have been forced underground, quietly meeting to minimize her weeping. If Dad and I aren't able to connect in the middle of the night, I pay attention to Mom's kitchen counter notes about various appointments, not only to remind Mom, but so I will know when Mom is gone and Dad's free. During days when Mom is home, Dad and I meet in parking lots, sitting in each other's car, savoring time connecting. Dad has become my main confidant and support. We talk about our pain in losing her and problem-solve the next exploding symptom or review symptoms already in progress. Sometimes during his lunch break, we go to a sub shop for a meal. But this is not our preference because our conversations are stunted in public—their nature too personal, too revealing, too emotional.

Opening the door to the dining room, heat rushes to envelop my body. Dad has been up awhile to have this room already cozy from the gas wall heater. Closing the door to the stairwell and living room, I hear Dad pouring tea water in the kitchen. Squinting in the bright light, Dad and I embrace. Inside his hug, I feel safe, peaceful and loved. I pick out my usual Sleepytime tea as spicy cinnamon wafts toward me from Dad's nearby mug.

Dad asks, "How did it go at the Alzheimer's support group?"

I'm glad he asks. It felt odd to sneak out of the house the other night so Mom wouldn't ask me where I was going.

"When I arrived at the group, they asked me if I was lost. I guess they didn't expect to see a 19-year-old at their meeting. I acted like I casually knew someone who has it but I didn't say anything about it being Mom. The meeting was geared toward people much older and more advanced than Mom, but the first-hand accounts of the advanced stages were hard to hear, especially thinking Mom will be there someday. Later in one of the discussions, they were shocked when I told them the person I know who has Alzheimer's disease is only 50 years old."

Dad listens with his squinty slate eyes energetically hugging me. His attention nearly brings me to tears.

I continue, "I'm not sure it was helpful, but it's nice to know there is an Alzheimer's support group nearby. If I were you, I wouldn't waste my time going right now, unless you need connection."

Dad stares down at his tea. It is not easy. I already know he needs more connection with other people for escape and to share the sorrow, but there is little extra time in his life beyond working and caring for Mom.

"Dad, how are you and Mom doing?"

Dad's stocky frame and curved shoulders push into his chair as his thick fingers rub the top lip of the ceramic mug. Steam swirls into the air.

A glossy film drips from his eyelids and crystal specks form on his cheeks. Tendons on each side of his neck tighten and his nostrils flare slightly as his soul begins to cry.

"Kate, it is so hard," he whispers, barely audible. "I'm losing my best friend. My heart breaks. She tries so hard and she means well. I don't know what else to do to help her."

Dad takes off his silver-rimmed bifocals and wipes his eyes before continuing. "The hardest part is when I'm sick or hurt. She used to ask me how I was feeling; now I have to tell her again and again that I'm not well. I try to hide my disappointment."

I reach across the table to hold his hand; he meets my hand halfway. With my free hand, I pass him a tissue, and then get a tissue for my own wet cheeks. Tears stream down his face. I'm grateful for our connection, but so sorry for his experience of emotional abandonment, isolation, loneliness, and sorrow.

"I love you. I'm so sorry," I say, at a total loss for any other words.

His free hand plays with his glasses that are folded into a triangle. A remaining teardrop melts off the glass lens and onto the table.

CHAPTER 7

✳

Can't Hide

AFTER COMPLETING MY SOPHOMORE year of college, I'm lifeguarding this summer and living at home. Mom has begun to admit her forgetfulness is more than emotional distress. She had been attributing it to the therapy sessions she was attending to deal with her sexually abusive childhood.

Sitting at the dining room table with Mom and Dad, we are eating spaghetti for the third night in a row. It has become common to have the same meals over and over, as Mom remembers something about pasta and decides that is a good choice for dinner. She prepares fresh pasta, even though leftovers are in green Tupperware in the fridge from the night before. Unwilling to make dinner every night, I bite my tongue. Despite the repetition, it is still yummy smothered in the homemade sauce that they canned last summer with tomatoes from Dad's garden.

Halfway through dinner, Mom says, "I forgot an important board meeting last night with the ambulance squad."

Dad asks, "What happened?"

"I dunno, I didn't write it down, I guess. Other members called me today to see why I didn't show up. I joked about it and asked them what I missed and how come they didn't invite me."

Then she adds, as if convincing herself, "It's not a big deal."

It's unusual for Mom to not attend a meeting, especially since she is the assistant chief. I have noticed Mom's forgetfulness is increasing and she continues to try and make up for it. Her humor is harsh and she jokes to cover up her mistakes.

Red sauce dries crimson on the dinner dishes that linger in front of us. I decide to let out one of the many questions I have been saving. "Mom, why don't you simply tell people that you have Alzheimer's?"

I don't realize the full impact of this question until Dad glances sternly at me and then reaches out his thick hand to touch Mom's arm. We both wait for her response.

Mom tenses, softening slightly to Dad's touch, and then declares, "I can't do that. It would ruin my life."

A tepid breeze blows through the open windows. I pause, listening but disagreeing. Then I respond, "Mom, I think it would benefit you. People would be more helpful and have more understanding when you forget something." Others would realize Mom isn't trying to be rude, mean, or bitchy; it is the disease getting in the way of how she normally communicates, but I don't dare tell her this.

"No, you don't understand. I won't even be able to walk down the street without someone picking me up and driving me home thinking that I'm lost."

Maybe she is right and I am selfish, tired of maintaining this secret. We, her family, are holding the secret, but she is an open book simply by how she relates with the world. There is no way to hide Alzheimer's disease.

I have watched the interactions that Mom has with the outside world. In the first five minutes she can hold her own with patterned conversations and habitual phrases. With or without being conscious of it, she has control of the subject matter, ensuring the other person doesn't talk about something she doesn't remember. However, after five minutes of talking to the same person, Mom begins to repeat once, twice, or more her familiar lines and conditioned responses.

Sometimes, though, Mom falls silent. This is easier for me, as I'm not embarrassed for her, yet it is sad, as Mom is no longer being herself and seems to be purposely hiding her failing skills.

Mom's face reddens and she reaches to gather the dirty dishes. I have pushed her too far tonight. Dad helps Mom bring them to the kitchen sink, and then he touches her arm gently. Mom turns into his waiting hug. I sit silent at the table and watch their love through the doorway between the dining room and kitchen. I fear things will never get better, but only grow worse, considering symptoms will increase. What does this mean for Dad?

I am deeply cut; sadness envelops me. I want someone to hold me and not say anything at all—especially not "It will be okay." Someone who will let me cry until all my sorrow is gone.

Bringing the remaining dishes to the kitchen, I tiptoe around their embrace.

CHAPTER 8

✳

Remarkable Patience

IT IS THREE A.M. Dad and I are sitting at our dining room table. This is the last summer I will spend lifeguarding. I've graduated with a multi-field major in environmental studies, sociology, and government. In the fall, Jim and I will enroll in an Adirondack AmeriCorps and Student Conservation Association program, teaching environmental education and doing trail work. I am 22.

"Dad, how do you do it? Mom is so annoying, demanding, and mean at times," I quiz him while warming my hands on my tea mug. Studying abroad in Kenya during this last year was a relief. I was engrossed in another culture away from home and Alzheimer's disease. Kenyans' stark fight for survival gave me an appreciation for my quality of life and my own luxury to worry about my family's future with Alzheimer's disease. Dad wrote me a letter nearly every day. When I was young, Mom used to write letters for both of them, but while I was on this trip, Mom just penned a few notes in simple sentences describing her daily activities. Halfway around the world, each letter brought fresh evidence of Mom's disease. I'm grateful to be close to Dad, but so sad to be losing Mom. Now, back at home, I struggle anew with how to accept and connect with her.

With a sparkle in his deep blues, Dad half-smiles and says, "I try to always remember that Mom's helping as she makes a ham sandwich when I asked for a veggie sandwich. The sandwich is still made with love. I want her to be herself and not paranoid, so I don't tell her when she forgets." His lemon tea steams and fogs his glasses as he carefully sips.

The Alzheimer's changes are creeping in fast and are difficult to see on a daily basis. I have less patience for the demands Mom is putting on Dad. *How does he find ways to enjoy what is left of their connection without becoming bitter and angry about all they have lost?*

Dad takes out a short article he keeps with him in his daily planner. He says, "I made a copy of this for you, too." He hands me the crisp sheet and I begin reading. It is about a husband who is caring for his wife who has Alzheimer's disease. She asks about her parents who died years before, and the husband patiently tells her they have passed away. After numerous explanations, the wife continues to question him about her parents. The husband, exhausted and angry, reaches a breaking point. Rummaging through the files to pull out the death certificates, he shoves the papers in front of his wife. She is now crying. The husband wishes he could take back his hasty, desperate action, but it is too late. He spends the night driving around the streets with his wife in the passenger seat, trying to help calm her until she drifts off to sleep, and the next day they will begin fresh again.

Examining his own wrinkled copy, Dad says, "I never want to do that to Maureen; it would crush her. Whenever I'm losing my patience, this story gives me the strength to continue caring for her in a loving manner."

✳

I'm sitting on the bed in Dad's office; he is shuffling papers at the desk. This was Dan's room before he moved to Oregon.

I say, "I don't know where to put my journals when I leave on trips. They are so important to me; I want them to be safe. Mom has no respect or sense of personal privacy anymore."

Dad nods without turning around. "What about storing them at a friend's house?"

I hate the fact that I can't trust my own mother. She is likely to take them to the dump thinking they are garbage. "What do you do with your journals?" I ask. Completely trusting Dad, I wonder about storing our journals together. In fact, he knows everything that they contain anyway.

"I destroyed all of them a couple of weeks ago."

I grab his arm, forcing him to look at me. "You destroyed them? Don't you want to re-read them? They tell your life's story. Why would you do that?"

Dad looks back at his desk. "I had to in case Mom accidentally came across them or if I die first. With Alzheimer's, she doesn't have the capacity to deal with anything negative she might read about our relationship or my feelings. No longer having the perspective to see the journal as events that happened in the past and that we were working through problems, she would dwell on the negative. I can't see any good that would come out of keeping them and I want to protect her from needless pain."

"So you don't write in a journal anymore?"

"I still write to get my thoughts down and to let go of anger, but now I destroy those sheets as soon as I write them."

Dad and I are sitting at the kitchen table. He is rubbing hand cream into his cracked hands.

Mom is still having headaches. She gets them whenever she is stressed. I say, "You are amazing with how much time you take massaging her head."

Dad shrugs and says, "I know the pain is real. I can feel the tension. As a machinist, my fingers learned sensitivity to subtle changes. I use that now when I massage the bones in Maureen's face and skull. I can feel when the headache breaks; as I hold the pressure points, I can sense the release."

Dad attributes that soothing touch as something he learned being a machinist, but I believe it is natural. When I would get sick as a little girl, he would put his warm hand on my head and pray for healing.

✳

Mom is making dinner and I'm sitting on the kitchen counter. Dad is putting ointment on his skin, and has been applying it for a couple of days.

I ask, "Dad, what is that for?"

"Mom and I have poison ivy."

I notice the slightest grin on his face, and he glances at Mom. She has been preoccupied by her own thoughts, but then quickly gets caught up to the conversation.

Dad says, "We think it is from Southwick's Beach."

It is my fourth summer working as a lifeguard at this beach. Curious, I ask, "Where did you guys go? Did you walk on the nature path?"

Mom says, "No, we went down the beach a-ways."

"It was growing right on the beach?" I ask.

At this point, Dad winks at Mom, and they communicate in their non-verbal language, which I can never understand. Something is amiss, but I don't know what it is.

"We went for a walk down the beach and then we wandered way off in the dunes to make love," Dad shyly confesses.

"What?" I ask in disbelief. This coming from my parents who never talk about "making love," and they are having sex in the open dunes? It takes me a while to process what I hear; then, I grin at how in love they both are, maybe more in love than ever.

Teenage smiles blaze across their aging, lined faces.

✳

CHAPTER 9

Lost Keys

THE YELLOWISH FORMICA KITCHEN counter is cool under my thighs. Leaning against the corner of the plywood cabinets, I'm deep in conversation with my sister-in-law Lori, who is visiting from Oregon. Lori's brown hair brushes her petite shoulders. With meekness and sincerity she asks honest, direct questions. I'm living at home, searching for a job after completing the Adirondack AmeriCorps program. Lori's legs swing freely on the opposite counter, her socked feet grazing the bottom cupboard. Mom has bustled through a couple of times, doing odd jobs and keeping herself busy. She is more comfortable on the move than in conversation. Taking all the keys off the rack, she inspects them and they clink together like coins.

"What are you looking for?" I ask.

"Dad's keys. He took my car and I can't find his key so I can run to the store." Putting on her lavender granny half-glasses that are hanging on the black rope around her neck, she peers again at the keys.

"Can I help?" I jump off the counter, sliding freely across the slippery floor, the way you can only do in front of family and good friends. I stop right in front of her and kiss her lightly on the cheek. The edge of her mouth turns the faintest bit upward.

"Hmmm … here it is, this silver one that is longer than the rest," I say.

"Where is the black one?"

"I don't know, but this one is the spare—it will work."

"Well, I will go see if it works," she says, bolting out the swinging door.

Two minutes later, Mom returns.

"What is wrong?" I ask again.

"I need the key for Dad's car."

Taking the keys from her, I ask, "Did you try this one?" pointing to the long silver key.

"Oh, no, I was looking for the black one."

I walk with Mom to the door. Her stocky frame hustles down the driveway. White hair tossing in the wind, I see her clutching the key between her thumb and index finger, the rest of the keys hanging loose.

Forty-five minutes pass and Lori motions to the clock. "Where is your mom?"

My muscles tighten and I catch my breath. Gaping at the clock, my mind races. *Where is Mom? Did her driving create an accident?* Then, I force myself to think rationally. I glance at the top of the fridge. The black walkie-talkie-sized scanner that monitors the local emergency services has been silent, so I know there hasn't been a serious accident.

Finally I say, "I don't know. I better go check on her. Getting milk usually doesn't take this long." I'm embarrassed that I was so engrossed in the conversation that I hadn't been the one to notice.

Pulling into the huge parking lot at Rod's Big M, I'm reminded of when Mom taught me how to slide the car around on snow and ice by pulling the emergency brake. Watching for light posts, I couldn't believe she really wanted me to pull the brake and turn the wheel. Mom insisted that I do it, especially because we lived in upstate New York. She had said, "This is how your car will handle in bad weather; you must be prepared for it and know how to steer out of it."

"Relax and enjoy the ride," echoes in my head.

I find Dad's navy Galant parked in the third slot in the middle row. I search for Mom. I see her, hunched and walking fast toward the store. Powering down the passenger side window, I yell, "Mom, Mom."

She stops, and turns around. She comes hustling over. "I can't find the key, maybe I lost it inside," she says, leaning on my car.

"Okay, I'm going to park and then I will help you." I pull ahead and park my red Galant three spaces away in the next open spot.

I jump out of the car, leaving the door ajar, and give Mom a hug. "Are you alright?"

"Yeah, just frustrated." She leans to the side to shove her hand into the opposite pocket to pull out the keys. "I had the key to get here. Maybe it fell off the ring."

"May I see the keys?" I ask, holding out my hand. "Mom, this is the key that works."

Mom takes the key, and, pressing her lips into a tight-lipped pucker she snickers, "Ooo, I didn't recognize it."

"I will meet you at home?" I ask.

"Yeah, thanks for coming to look for me."

I touch my heart as I watch her drive past my parking spot. Taking a deep breath and straightening my spine, I put my car in reverse and then follow her for the one and a half miles to our home. Feeling like a helpless parent of a kindergartner, I watch her every move, wanting her to be protected, at peace, and have help whenever needed.

CHAPTER 10

Bamboozled

SHARP CORNERS OF THE large metal desk are outlined by the powder blue walls of Dad's office. Amber fall light pours through the window onto his desk, illuminating his large hands holding open a manila folder. He is skimming notes and numbers through his bifocals. His normally squinty, happy eyes are wide with distress and his thick lips are pressed together.

"I don't see another way. Paying for Mom's supplements and vitamins as well as the specialists that are not covered by insurance is expensive. We have already refinanced the house. There is nothing left." Dad continues to shuffle papers from various financial advisors and debt counselors. "I have to file for bankruptcy."

My spirit aches as I watch his ideological values collide with daily reality.

Mom has been applying for various jobs, but has been unsuccessful. Six months ago she lost her job as a courier for a medical company when it restructured. She tried USPS rural routes but wasn't able to perform basic skills. She began working for UPS in Liverpool, an hour away. Dad and Mom went together on the first day. On the second day, Mom, who used to have an exceptional sense of direction, couldn't find the UPS building. Lost and crying, she called Dad. Mom, although disappointed in yet another loss, exclaimed, "Well, at least I was paid for one day of work."

Volunteering at the rescue squad is also at stake, as one by one Mom is losing her medical certifications. She is able to do the practical tests, but she isn't able to successfully translate her skills onto a written exam. The members of the ambulance squad have kindly requested her to stay involved by driving the ambulance or assisting in the back. I'm not sure she has officially told them about Alzheimer's disease, but they must suspect something is wrong.

Dad sets the paperwork on the faux wood desktop. "I want to talk with all of you kids about it first. How do you feel if I go bankrupt?"

"Dad, it's not really your fault. You didn't try to screw over anyone. You have been helping Mom; you haven't been wasteful. Any money mismanagement was from Mom's Alzheimer's disease and we have stopped most of that."

Last month, I spent hours on the phone with *Reader's Digest* canceling Mom's subscription. Initially, I called to cancel the large-print edition we were receiving in addition to the standard font edition, when I realized the much bigger problem of prepaid subscriptions for nine years into the future. Every time they sent a bill or notice to renew for a cheap price, Mom would send off a check. She thought she was getting a deal and was afraid the subscription would run out if she didn't mail a check immediately.

A door-to-door salesman bamboozled Mom with a water refiner for $4,000. He didn't know she was ill—in short interactions she appears mentally competent. She agreed to purchase it without the usual discussion with Dad. Dad felt obligated to go ahead with it, even when I told him that legally he wasn't bound. Dad felt stuck in the middle between stepping on her ego and her desire for soft water versus asserting what they could afford. All the while, he was also confronting the emotional pain of the relationship change in decision making. No longer could decisions be mutual; he would make them and then talk with Mom until she understood and felt like they had made the decision together.

"Dad, I don't care if you file for bankruptcy, especially if it will ease your mind in any way."

"I hate that I can't pay my bills. I mean to honor every debt we have had, buhht … " his voice trails off. The knuckles of his first two fingers are pinching the end of his nose as he brings his lips up to touch them.

"If only I can get the hang of driving the milk truck by myself and backing up at all the different farms; that will bring in more money and Maureen can come with me," Dad says, rubbing his temples with the pointer finger and thumb of his right hand. He reclines in the chair with his toes pushing off the ground. "What I really need is to be home with her during the day. I think I will be able to work only half time as an auditor—I have already mentioned this to my boss. I love the work, but Maureen needs me. The last specialist we saw encouraged us to enjoy the time we have left, as she is slipping fast."

"Dad, are you taking care of yourself, exercising and taking time for you?" I ask, glimpsing his taut pot belly pushing against his t-shirt.

"I'm walking a couple of times a week with Mom. That has been good. The other day, my peripheral vision got blurry and I could only see straight ahead. I have also had some chest pain lately."

"Did you go the doctor? You know that could be a sign of more serious stuff like a heart attack or stroke."

"I went to the doctor's three weeks ago and he gave me a full physical."

"So what did you do when your vision became blurry?"

"I lay down for a bit to relax and I was fine when I got up."

"How do you feel now? Don't you think you should get checked?"

"I feel fine. I did a physical stress test at the doctor's and with the clean bill of health, I must be okay."

Offhandedly he says, "I need to keep my stress down."

I laugh at Dad as I shrug and nod toward the desk. *Did he really say that nonchalantly?*

Dad suddenly sees the absurdity of it himself and he bursts into laughter. His fiercely independent wife has Alzheimer's. Finances are strapped. He is working two jobs and caring for her. He thinks he can easily lower his stress level. Holding his belly, tears roll down his face, and he chuckles, "Ooo, ooo, that is funny."

CHAPTER 11

❋

Guilt for Leaving

"ARE YOU WILLING TO make a two-year commitment?" one of the five interviewers on the conference call interrogates me over the phone. If I get this job, I will be a community organizer for a social and environmental justice organization located in Kentucky. I've been out of college for two years; I am 24. My mind races and I proceed cautiously, watching my words.

"Yes. I'm excited about this job; it's my dream job and matches my self-sculpted major perfectly." Nervousness cuts my words as the tone moves uncontrollably from hope to fear, high to low. The rest of the conversation is a blur, filled with *thanks for the interview* and *we will get back to you*. And then the hard *click*, as I hang up the phone.

After reaching for my journal, I retreat into a semi-fetal position, cradling my résumé and notes in front of me. The words I scrawl are jagged with passionate ink. *They never directly asked me. Of course I would leave if anything happens.*

Bbring…startled, I jump up. *Bbring*…I grab a tissue, and dry my face and blot my nose. *Bbring … Uhhmmm*, I clear my throat. Taking a deep breath, I answer the phone.

"Kate, we would like to invite you for a personal interview."

"Uhhhhh, Jerry, I'm glad you called. There's something that I want you to be aware of." My voice is already shaking. "My mother has early-onset Alzheimer's disease. It shouldn't impact my work in any way, but I wanted you to know my whole situation."

"Thanks for telling me, we understand extenuating circumstances may arise," Jerry tells me kindly. Nothing more is said about that and we go on to discuss scheduling the interview. Another *click*; this one is soft.

I jump up, suspended in air with both arms overhead, shouting, "Yes, I did it, they want me! They like me!" I wiggle my hips from side to side, shifting the weight on my feet, then, pulling one knee at a time to my chest, I march exaggerated across the floor. Everything is lighter; my body floats to the mirrored bathroom door and without thinking, I kiss the cold glass reflection before laughing out loud as I run and somersault onto the fluffy, pearl-colored down comforter stretched across the bed.

It has been one month since the phone interview, and two weeks ago I traveled to Kentucky. They offered me the job and I accepted it. Meanwhile, back at home, my boyfriend Jim's stepfather, Buz, had a heart attack. I'm cat- and house-sitting for Buz and Carol, Jim's mom, while they are staying at St. Joseph's Hospital in Syracuse.

Leaving their house, I drive to Rod's Big M to find boxes to pack for my move to Kentucky where my new job awaits me. Speeding up Main Street, I peer out the passenger side window as I pass my family's white house with steel blue trim. The siding needs to be washed. It's dingy, but the American flag hanging off the porch billows proudly in the wind. Putting up and taking down the flag has become a task Mom utilizes to fill the space in her empty hours.

The electric doors of the grocery store swing open above the black grooved mat. The cardboard is kept in the back through the "employee only" rubber-lined aluminum doors. This morning when I called the store manager to request that they save some boxes for me, he told me to help myself. I stack the boxes one inside the other, keeping the ones with the easy handles, clean bottoms, and sturdy sides. I push aside the smelly egg and dairy cartons. Maneuvering backwards, I press against the doors and walk into the sprawling, brightly lit market. Boxes three in height with eight hidden, I crane my neck to the side, peering down the aisle in front of me.

"Hey, can I help?" an unmistakably familiar voice enthusiastically offers. I can't see her; the cardboard containers are in the way.

"Hi Mom, yeah, you can grab the top set," I say appreciatively. She snatches them, nearly skipping by my side as I walk along.

"What are you doing here?" I ask in the freezer section. Her hands were empty before taking the cardboard and there is no cart nearby.

"I saw you drive by, so I jumped in my car to follow you," she explains cheerfully.

I swallow hard. In a serious tone I ask, "Where were you?"

"I was in my bedroom and looked out my window as you drove by. I waved, but you didn't notice me."

The synchronistic joy inside of me fades. I want to grab those boxes out of her hands and tell her to leave me alone. I feel stalked by a mother who is behaving like a clingy 4-year-old sister. *Will I have to change routes to go from Buz and Carol's house to the grocery store?*

✳

I dial six numbers: 232-303—then, *click*, hit the off button on the black cordless phone. I glance at the clock on the wall, out the window, and return to the keypad. Again, I press the same six numbers, and again follow with a click. I put the phone down on the glass table and get a drink of water from Buz and Carol's kitchen.

Soon I will be leaving for Kentucky, where I see a glimmer of hope, escape, and a chance to feel the buried anger and sadness that boils within me. And perhaps these poisonous feelings will dissipate with time and distance. But with thoughts of freedom come waves of guilt. I'm terrified to leave. *What will Dad do? Will he ask for help? We will still talk and cry on the phone, but who will hug him with understanding? Mom asks me for help; who will she call when she needs a key, a hug, or something to do? How can I possibly leave them? How can I possibly stay without part of me shriveling up to die?*

I grab the phone and quickly dial the seven digits before I can change my mind. It rings twice; every hair on my arms is standing upright. I wait, not breathing. I called last night, but ended up talking in circles with Mom for fifteen minutes.

"Hello," Dad's voice answers.

"Ahhh. Hi Dad, it's Kate—but wait, I don't want you to put Mom on the line. I would like to talk with only you."

"Hi Kate," he begins. I cringe, waiting. Mom always picks up the other phone when she knows it is me. He continues, "She's at a meeting tonight."

I breathe again, deeper, filling my lungs. We will not have to talk in code.

"I've been thinking about our conversation from the other day and have a few suggestions that I would like to help put in place before I leave for Kentucky to make it easier on you."

"I would like to hear what you are thinking," he says in a slow, quiet voice. His tone sounds open to what I have to say, but his words bother me. It's as if he will listen to me, but won't act on my suggestions.

"People in the community have offered to help, and I think we should ask for meals to be delivered a couple of times a week. I will call and arrange it and then ask one of them to organize it when I'm gone."

"That is a good idea, but we are not ready for it yet. Maureen is still trying to make some meals. I don't want to discourage her attempts."

"Alright. What about asking them to stop over during the day to be sure Mom is okay, the stove is off, the windows are not open with the heat on—all the stuff you do when you come home? Mom wouldn't even have to know they are checking up on her. They could arrange to come over for a cup of tea or bring lunch. This way Mom would still have interaction, you would know she was safe, and you could use that time for yourself."

"I want to be the one to do that. I schedule my audits around home and stop by about twice a day." His voice is solid and de-termined.

"Dad, are you sure? Is there anything that I can help you with before I leave?" I ask. I wish Dad would accept help, but I know I can't force my wishes on him and Mom. It is their life. I can make suggestions, but then I must let go.

"No, but thanks for the offer. You have done more than enough already. Thanks for staying around so long, it has been a treat. We will be fine, we will miss you terribly, but it is important for you to do this. We know you will do well and are excited for you."

I cry after hanging up the phone, I feel so helpless and angry; I want to fix the situation. If I stay, I get consumed with either my own anger at the toll this disease is taking on Dad or my sorrow over losing Mom. I do know Dad means everything he said on the phone. However, I feel guilty leaving them and guilty staying with my negative emotions. I'm giving up on my life if I stay. I'm abandoning family need or responsibility if I leave.

CHAPTER 12

Ominous Reality

I WAKE SWEATING AND disoriented with a heavy boulder lying on my chest. I am struggling for air. A sharp edge, like an arrowhead, sears deep, stabbing all the way into my spine, etching unknown markings into my ivory bones. I stumble to the gunmetal-gray heater and yank the cord from the wall. Ripping off my damp clothes, I lay naked on top of the thick covers in the dark room.

My mind is foggy, as if in an altered state. I rub my chest for the next hour, trying to get the pain to subside. I'm aware there is no phone easily accessible in this abandoned brick dormitory in London, Kentucky. Who would I call anyway? Dad? What would I say?

Awakening in the morning, there are robins playing gleefully together outside. In the shower, I feel the vibration of "Amazing Grace." Usually I disown this religious part of my history, but today as I sing, I don't mind it echoing against the slick ceramic tiles. Toweling off, I put a drop of delicate rose oil on my sternum. It will help the pain that still throbs inside. The rich, sweet scent explodes inside my nose, ears, and throat.

Taking one last glimpse around the room before I walk to

work, my gaze is drawn to my healing stones. Spontaneously, I carefully tuck them one by one into my pocket. Like a two-year-old gathering rocks, I have no explanation for why, today, these stones seem important. They have been given to me by various significant people in my life—good friends, a yoga teacher, a counselor—or I have gathered them from my favorite locations.

Stepping outside to walk the block and a half from my temporary dorm housing to my job, the sun beats down between fluffy white clouds, and fifteen iridescent black crows jump and fly along beside me. A few peck at the dirt.

My desk is nestled at the top of the stairs. *Call Lamar* is written on a yellow Post-It note inside a navy three-ring welcome binder, along with a list of duties for my orientation week. Burt, my supervisor, fit and handsome with his brown hair, trimmed beard, and smile lines that caress his facial features, climbs the stairs two at a time.

He greets me. "Good morning. Your brother—or maybe it was your brother-in-law—called this morning and asked for you to call one of your siblings."

"Thanks for the message," I reply. "Are you available to go over the schedule for this week? I have a couple of questions."

"Yeah, but it sounds to me like you should call your siblings first," he replies.

Quizzically, I watch him walk into his office. I feel like he is pushing it on me, which seems unusual for him, despite the short time I have known him.

The large beige desk phone is flashing red on lines one and three. I pull out my long-distance calling card and proceed to dutifully dial the numbers. It is too early in Oregon to call Dan or Jay. I will try my sister Karen in New Hampshire. As the phone begins to ring, I flip through the welcome binder and my eyes settle on the recommended reading list.

"Hi Guy, it's Kate."

"Hi Kate. Hold on, I'll get Karen." His voice is strained. Surprised by the curt conversation, I close the binder and sit up straight in my chair. *What is going on? Something must have happened with Mom—did she burn down the house or get in an accident?* I scan the deserted playground across the street, noticing dark clouds are forming shadows on the ground.

I hear Karen sniffling in the background. My breath quickens as I strain my ears and push the phone squarely into the side of my head. Guy whispers to her, "Hon, it's Kate." I hear the phone changing hands.

"*Ff-ff-ffsz,*" Karen sniffs into the phone, "*Nnnnhuha-a-a,* Kkate." In my mind I can see her brown hair, glasses, and her sad face, but I've never heard her voice hyperventilate. "Dddddaaadd Ddddi-ah-ah-ie-ied." She breaks into sobs.

"Wha-What? Dad died? You mean Mom, right? Not Dad," I implore.

"No-oh, Kkate, Ddahd Diheed." My body convulses in terror and my eyes stare blindly out the window.

I have only been gone a week. Guilt and pain cruise through my body, bottlenecking in my throat. *RRRKrraackk.* Red lightning explodes from the dark cloud that hovers over the phone. Striking. My soul fragments. It is exposed and sprawled out with no hope of recovery.

Roseann, one of my co-workers, hears my sobs. I write in shaky letters on the big sheet of paper in front of me *My Dad— Dead*. She gasps, "Oh, Dear Lord," touching the base of my neck, and she says a quick prayer for me.

Last night I watched *Tuesdays with Morrie* at her house and we had talked about how close Dad and I had become through Mom's Alzheimer's disease.

She had asked in her Southern accent, "How can your parents stand to let you go this far away? They must miss you terribly."

That evening, sitting in the Syracuse airport parking lot, Jim, my boyfriend of seven years, and I hold each other, crying.

"How did you find out?" I ask.

"Dan called and woke me this morning and asked me to 'find out what the hell was going on.' Todd had called Dan to tell him Dick was going to the hospital in the ambulance and they were doing CPR. Todd and Maureen were at the hospital and I drove there to see what was happening."

Todd's house is less than a block away from Mom and Dad, down the back hill and across the baseball diamond of the elementary school.

I ask Jim, "What did he look like?" referring to my dad.

"You don't really want me to tell you, do you?" he asks, concerned.

"Yeah, Jim, I have to know it all," I say, touching his thick arm hair.

"Well, I was in the hospital with your mom, and someone recognized me as a respiratory therapist and asked if I knew Dick Preskenis. When I told them yes, they asked me to do the identification of him in the morgue." Jim pauses, swallowing hard. "It was eerie. When the doctor pulled back the sheet, the face was ashen, gray-blue. It was your father, but he was vacant." Jim's eyes fill and begin to glisten. "I verified it was him. Kate, it was the hardest thing I have ever done."

We pull into the driveway, the very one I left days prior with my car packed. Karen rushes out to see me and we fall together in a desperate hug, our abdomens heaving as we wail in unison. Our bodies fit together perfectly, and we hold each other tighter than ever.

Our hug is interrupted when Mom swings open the door. Her wild white hair is as erratic as her movements.

Mom wraps me in a bear hug and cries, "Oh Katie, I'm so sorry for you. You were so close to him. Oh, what will we do?" At Mom's first grasp, I try to quit crying so I can be strong and console her. Then I realize it is fruitless.

Stunned by her recognition of my pain in the midst of her own, I say, "I'm sorry too, Mom. I love you." Trembling, she is out of breath; her insides are going one hundred miles per hour. I recognize that loose cannon rumble.

She wonders aloud, "What will I do without Dick?"

I wonder how long Mom will remember that Dad has died.

Our embrace loosens. The whites of her eyes are bloodshot and her nose is raw from crying. Then I notice her dreadful, morbid, dark-bruised lips from giving Dad mouth to mouth. This is the most gripping, ominous sign of the day's reality.

I want to go to the morgue to see Dad, but am afraid to go alone. No one else seems interested and I fear it will haunt me forever. Where is Dad's soul, is it here in the house where he died? Is it over his body? Is it with each one of us? Is it in "heaven?" I want to see him NOW; I don't want to wait until the funeral.

Lingering awake, despite my heavy eyelids that match the weight of my heart, I sneak to the same spot where Dad died. Taking a worn patchwork quilt from inside the coat closet at the base of the stairs, I lie down on the floor on the stairs' landing. A small night light illuminates the golden hardwood that is stiff and cold under my body. I inspect the fancy wood-framed ceiling that Mom has painted baby blue and navy, each piece of trim a different color. The walls ascend with the stairs in a slick peach paint. Our yard light shines through the white double windows at the top of the stairs. Dad lay here eighteen hours ago. What was he thinking? Was he in pain? Did he know it was coming or did it take him by surprise? Did my leaving contribute to his death? I hate that he died alone, while Mom was on an ambulance call, while I was in Kentucky.

Curling into the fetal position, I feel crazy lying on the landing, but want to sleep here. However, realizing it may disturb Mom if she wakes to another person lying at the base of the stairs, I force myself to return to my bed, praying Dad will visit my dreams.

✳

CHAPTER 13

Tissue Box

IT'S THE NIGHT AFTER Dad died. Our house is swarming with at least thirty relatives. Everyone is restless and busy—looking at photo albums, talking about "Dick," making food, washing dishes, finishing funeral plans, calling people to inform them of Dad's death and doting on Mom—as if by being busy they might fix this absolutely unfixable situation.

Agitated, tense, hot, I want to get out of here. My head feels like it's going to explode from grief and surges of anger. No matter how much I love them, being surrounded with all these chattering and crying people doesn't give me the distraction I long for. After telling my siblings that I'm going to visit Jim, I purposefully move through the kitchen and wait impatiently near the door, seeking the opportune time to sneak away from Mom. She has become glued, as tight as a shadow, to us kids since Dad died. I can't deal with Alzheimer's tonight.

I grab my jacket and Dad's car keys and step outside into the refreshing, nearly winter air. The coolness dries my sweat from the heat of the crowded house. I walk past two coolers under the kitchen window overflowing with gifts of food from neighbors and friends.

The navy Galant is in the driveway where Dad had parked it the night before. He pulled straight in, rather than his characteristic backing-in parking style. It smells like Dad's car: traces of lemon tea, lots of paperwork, and carbon paper. The car feels familiar, so much like Dad; how can he be gone? I sit in the driver's seat and shut the door. Looking at the tissue box on the passenger seat, I put my forehead to the steering wheel, searching my body for the strength to drive. My heart hurts. My knees are weak. I haven't driven since Dad died. I can't see through my tears.

Getting out of the car, fresh air greets my lungs again as my breath staggers. The stars show beyond the yard light attached to the garage and I wonder if Dad is somewhere out there. I hope he is still here, but how can anyone really know about the other side from this one? His garden is now barren. I remember he took pleasure in growing vegetables, but mostly he loved planting strawberries for his grandkids. He worked the soil and I would sit on the grass and watch. He never seemed to mind that I rarely helped; he was glad for my company.

I turn to view the extended family bustling about inside the glowing glass of the house. Mom moves in the yellow, picture-framed dining room window and then walks off to the right. I watch the kitchen window where she reemerges into the brighter white florescent lighting. Her head is down; she is looking for something. From one room to the next, I watch as if it's a TV screen. Fake, distant, yet captivating.

Gathering my energy, I return to the car, determined to drive away. I climb in the car and recoil, startled. The tissue box is now sitting in the middle console between the two front seats, right where it usually sat when Dad and I would spend time together. We often grieved and the tissues were a constant third companion to our talks. Am I imagining the original placement of the tissues on the seat? No, I distinctly remember them there, and I never touched them. I never reached beyond this seat before I got out.

"Dad?" my voice quivers as chills ripple through my body, "Are you here? Did you move the tissues because we are both here?"

CHAPTER 14

Aftermath

"HOLD ON, START OVER. What happened? It doesn't make sense," I quiz Todd. We are standing in the living room with the glass door shut, securing privacy from others in the rest of the house. It is mid afternoon, a day before Dad's funeral. Through the windows I see vehicles drive up and down Main Street under the dreary gray sky.

"South Jefferson Rescue Squad had a call in the middle of the night," Todd patiently describes the night Dad died. Earlier this week, Todd briefly told me his version of the incidents surrounding Dad's death. I've asked to talk with him again to try to understand.

I persist. "But I thought Mom quit taking volunteer calls without Dad, and they both decided to stop taking calls during the night because Dad had to work during the day."

"Over the scanner the rescue squad called for additional help to assist with lifting the patient, so I guess your parents decided to help. They needed manpower, as a huge guy was having a heart attack on the third floor of the Hotel Adams. There is no elevator, so the ambulance crew had to carry him down three flights of stairs on a stretcher."

Todd continues, "Afterward, Mo went to the hospital in the ambulance. Dick went home. The last interaction he had was with a firefighter who also helped carry the man down the stairs. I've talked to that firefighter; he said Dick seemed fine. They had a normal conversation and Dick never let on he was in any pain.

"Then, I heard another call come over the scanner. Help was needed here at this address. I didn't bother with my Jeep; I just ran up the back hill and was the first one on the scene, other than your mom. Your dad was lying on the floor at the base of the stairs."

"Did it look like he fell? What was Mom doing?" I ask.

"No, it didn't appear to be a fall; he had an arm propped under his head like he was resting. Your mom was freaking out; she had found him when she returned from the first ambulance call. I told her we had to start CPR and began to coach her through it, telling her when to give the rescue breaths as I was doing chest compressions."

"Didn't she remember on her own after all those years on the squad?"

"She wasn't doing it when I arrived."

"Was he still alive when you arrived?"

Todd paused. "No, to me he was obviously gone. If I had arrived on the scene in any other situation, I would never have started CPR. But for Dick, I had to. I would have never forgiven myself."

I trust Todd's evaluation of the scene not only because he is my brother, but also because he is a police officer and volunteer firefighter. We met Todd through a Mennonite church when I was in junior high school. Dan and Todd were friends and Todd's foster home was not a good situation, so after a family discussion, we asked Todd if he wanted to live with us and be part of our family. I'm not sure what happened to his parents, but I know he lived with his grandfather and one day found his grandfather dead. Todd was in elementary school. It was then that he entered the foster care system. I hate that he also saw my dad's dead body, too.

"What else happened?"

"They took Dick to the hospital in the ambulance. Then I called Dan and I stayed with your mom."

Quieter now, I muse, "So Dad died of a massive heart attack after helping another heart attack victim?"

"Yeah."

Did that man live?
Does it matter?

I wander the house aimlessly. Food, sleep, and journal writing have been replaced with basic survival: Breath. Water. Hugs. The pain in my chest has alarmed my siblings, but I think it is emotion, along with the boil that popped up on my hand and the constant burning in my lungs.

It has been one week since Dad died. I go into Mom and Dad's room about three times a day to open his drawers, look at his clothes, and smell his lingering scent.

We had a policy growing up that no one was allowed to go into another's room, never mind dresser drawers, without permission. Now, Dad is dead and I'm sneaking into his room searching for some solace. Afraid to ask for Mom's consent in all her Alzheimer's disease confusion and grief, I tiptoe to the tall, thin dresser when she is downstairs.

Taking a cotton T-shirt out of his drawer, I bring it to my face. On first inhale, it smells mostly of Era detergent, but on the second inhale there is a thin veil of perspiration and a hint of sweet honey. His essence is gold to this aching heart.

Burying my face in his pillow, I breathe in deep. There is the other indescribable human scent of his scalp, uniquely associated with love and safety. It curls up my nostrils into my brain and circles down toward my abdomen. *Ah, this is how he smelled when we hugged.*

I take two full breaths before I have to quickly move away from it so I don't dilute the smell with my weeping. Ritualistically returning it to rest flush with Mom's pillow, I pick up the T-shirt.

All of a sudden, my neck tightens as I feel someone nearby. I turn around slowly. Standing in the doorway, Mom's cold, protruding stare rotates from me to the open dresser drawer and back again.

Red-hot hands hold the white Hanes V-neck T-shirt inches from my face, while cool blue blood drains to my lead feet. *How did she sneak up those squeaky stairs without my hearing?* Bracing myself, I watch her as another salty drop coagulates on my eyelash and is slowly lowered to my cheek.

Her alarm turns to compassion when she sees the tear touch my cheek. "Kate, you can take that shirt. Is there anything else that you want?"

How does Alzheimer's drive most of Mom's interactions, and then suddenly Alzheimer's is gone and it is my mom again? Is there any physical thing that I want? Nothing physical will fill this emotional loss. And then I want everything, so I never forget him even for a second. Like Bob, who wore Dad's tie, shirt, pants, underwear, and socks at the funeral; everything seems sacred.

Mom is standing in the doorway, concern in her eyes, waiting for me to answer. She would give me anything.

Is there anything else I want? Yeah, I want Dad back. And I want you back—How did Alzheimer's loosen its grip right now? I'm sobbing for the loss of Dad, but more for the surprising and refreshing presence of Mom.

Mom walks to me. I rise from the bed. Throwing her arms around me, she bear-hugs me. *Mom, how did you break through the Alzheimer's tangles? Will you stay here mentally, present emotionally, please—like a trade? Dad is already gone, but you get to come back fully?*

I need you. I need someone. I can't believe you are comforting me. I feel guilty; I should be comforting you. Where is your grief?

Bbzzzzzzzzzzzzzzzzzzz. ... the dull sound grows louder as I approach the cellar. Walking down the wooden stairs, I see that Mom has one foot on top of a five-gallon bucket to stabilize an eight-foot-long board. She has one hand on the circular power saw and the other on the two-by-four. *Bbzzzzzzzzz.*

"Ma," I yell.

Bbzzzzzzzzz. "Ma, be careful," I scream. My normally safe mom is reckless, her body off balance.

When the electrical whizzing stops, I ask, "Why did you take that off?" referring to the saw's safety guard that is lying on the ground.

"Ah, it always gets in the way."

"May I hold the board for you?" I ask, but don't feel safe myself with her hand barely controlling the heavy, awkward spinning saw.

Bbzzzzzzzz. I hadn't thought of it before, but safety with power tools is one more issue my siblings and I have to address, especially since carpentry work is familiar to her.

Sitting on the floor in Buz and Carol's living room, Jim and

I are putting together small black lanterns that are solar powered and will light their front walkway. The yard lights were bought today from Sam's Club. Their kitchen, dining room, and living room are open, essentially one large L-shaped room. I can hear Carol clinking dishes at the sink. Ever since Dad died, I feel attached to Buz, as if I can somehow experience part of Dad's final hour through the stories of Buz's heart attack.

Tactful and tentative, Buz sits awkwardly in the plush La-Z-Boy chair, as if he were resting on an uncomfortable, bumpy, and sloped tree stump. When he gets up, he moves slowly, balancing on the strength of his forearm until he can get his legs positioned underneath him. Buz drinks a lot of fluid. Baggy gray sweatpants cover the thigh incision from the graft that was taken for his quadruple bypass. As he limps to the bathroom, he says the leg incision is more painful than his chest.

Returning again to the recliner with the black massage pad, Buz sits down gingerly. A tiny silver time capsule on a chain around his neck contains nitroglycerin, miracle medicine to calm the ticking bomb, his heart, and carry him through until he reaches the hospital if another attack grips his body.

"Buz, will you tell me about your heart attack?" I ask, snapping a black hood over a clear plastic lantern.

"I got up from the hospital staff meeting and took up my food tray," Buz begins. "I felt a little tightness; I thought it was indigestion. I fell down, but I don't remember that part. I was lucky to be in the hospital. My co-workers started CPR right away.

"The next thing I remember, my sisters were greeting me and I was at peace and didn't have any pain. Then, a while later, my sisters were gone and Carol was standing over me. I tried to speak, but it was garbled. I managed to stammer, 'Are my sisters here?' Carol was concerned, but steadfast. She didn't respond. I asked again, 'Are my sisters alive?' Carol said, 'No, both of your sisters have passed away.'"

Goosebumps hopscotch across my body. Buz goes on, "I wouldn't be concerned about your father; he is in a better place. I have confidence in that. It was peaceful and beautiful, like they say; the light was warm and comforting. He is surrounded by people who love him."

Tears stream down my face and I have to keep blowing my nose. I can't stop blubbering even when I try. I was crying during dinner after hearing Carol say grace. Buz and Carol tried to ignore it and go on with conversation. Jim touched my knee soothingly under the table and that brought fresh tears. I had to direct all my focus onto the food. Mashed potatoes: put on fork, bring to mouth, bite, chew, and swallow.

With a slight sheen over his eyes, Buz continues softly, "Your dad and mom visited us here days before he died. Carol and I tried to get them to come inside, but they didn't want to be guests, or to wear us out as we were returning from the hospital. They stopped to see if we needed anything and to wish us well." Buz raises his salt and pepper eyebrows, then looks down and off to the right. Carol leaves the dishes to sit near Buz. She kneels next to his chair, her strong, steady, tan hand on his armrest.

"Dick told me he was glad I was alive." The sheen breaks as three drops trickle down his face. He wipes them with the back of his thick, muscular hand. His upper lip quivers as he continues. "I don't understand why your father died and I lived. That is something I struggle with daily," he says with a one-shoulder shrug. "I guess I'm not through here."

CHAPTER 15

Oregon or Bust

DAN, BOB, AND MOM are tightly packed into the front seat of the orange U-Haul cab. After already enduring the loss of his birth mother, Bob is now coping with the gradual decline of his adopted mom (oldest sister) along with the sudden loss of Dad, his adopted father. Now, side by side, they are nearly as close as three months ago when Bob tenderly cuddled Mom to sleep in the nights immediately following Dad's death.

All of Mom and Dad's furniture, clothes, bedding, and miscellaneous items are in the rear of the U-Haul. Not much is worth saving, except that it is familiar to Mom. Oregon is the place where most of the siblings agreed we could both care for her long term and find employment. Dan and Jay are already established there, Karen moved six weeks ago, and when I leave Kentucky, I will join them. The first attempt to get Mom to Oregon was when Karen moved, but on the morning of the move Mom backed out, saying she didn't want to leave New York. After a failed second attempt three weeks ago, we decided to leave Mom alone in New York and have her friends check on her, but not provide her with constant company. We were trying to facilitate her decision to be surrounded by her children. This is the third attempt to move

Mom to Oregon; she wants to be with her kids but doesn't want to surrender her life in Adams.

Immediately after cramming into the cab of the U-Haul, Dan hands Mom the essential items to keep her occupied: a caffeine-free Diet Pepsi, a roll of Butter Rum Life Savers, her water bottle, and a *Reader's Digest* with her reading glasses. The U-Haul eases out of the driveway, towing Mom's Toyota Corolla behind. Then Dan heads as fast as possible to Route 81 southbound before Mom can change her mind again.

A few miles down the road, upon passing the first rectangular sign that advertises a restroom, Mom says, "Let's stop."

"You used the bathroom right before we left," Bob exclaims.

"I have to go again," she states without hesitation.

They reluctantly stop. After using the facilities, Mom reaches into her pocket, pulls out change, and inserts it into the vending machine. Wielding a Diet Pepsi, Mom climbs into the cab.

As Dan begins to pull onto the highway, Bob says, "Get this thing up to speed so we don't get run over."

"I am; this thing is floored," Dan explains.

"Well, drive in the breakdown lane till we get it going."

"Oh, right, and hit some pothole that pops a tire? You want to drive this thing? Because I will pull over right now and you can take over," Dan half offers, half threatens.

Bob raises his hand. "No, I don't want to drive, relax. I was making a suggestion. It wasn't criticism."

Within twenty minutes, Mom says, "Hey, when you see a bathroom, pull over, will you? I've gotta go."

Dan and Bob look at the second empty Diet Pepsi bottle in her hands. She always chooses a bottle, because "Cans are made of aluminum and that contributes to Alzheimer's." It's always diet "Sugar isn't good for you." She insists on caffeine-free "So it doesn't keep me up at night."

Dan simply says, "Sure Mom, no problem."

Bob's commentary about Dan's driving subsides. They stop at the next rest area and thereafter attempt to keep drinks away from Mom and distract her from seeing the restroom signs.

Two full days of traveling have passed. Bob can't bear being crammed in the front seat any longer with Mom constantly asking, "Where are we going? How much longer? Where are we going?" Finally, he makes a bed in the storage area of the U-Haul and crawls inside, pulling down the sliding door behind him.

Several hours later, while driving from Denver on Route 25 towards Cheyenne, people in passing cars stare purposefully into the cab. Dan looks at them with his blonde Abe Lincoln beard, raising his hands, and says, "What?!?" Then, he continues driving like normal, cruising down the road at 75 mph. Mom is asleep in the passenger seat. Finally, he gets to enjoy the song that has been on his mind since he left Oregon to be with Mom: John Denver's "Take Me Home, Country Roads."

Loud honking interrupts his peace. Another driver is wagging his finger out the window toward the rear of the truck. Dan searches the side mirrors, and even winds down the window, but doesn't see anything. Tires seem to be fine, car is still on the trailer, no police lights; no problem.

Meanwhile, Bob has lifted the tailgate, precariously exposing Mom's belongings. The potholes and bumps threaten to scatter them across the bumpy Colorado highway. He waves a pillow case, trying to get Dan's attention. After ten minutes with no response, Bob rummages through the items until he finds a ski pole onto which he attaches the white fabric. Bracing himself in the doorway, holding on with one arm, he waves the flag up and down, hoping to get Dan's attention. Bob's long, blonde curly hair flies in all directions like a madman's.

A mile or two later, Dan sees something flashing in the side mirror. It's the white truce flag.

Stopping at the next rest area, Bob jumps out yelling, "I didn't think you were ever going to stop! I've been trying to get your attention ever since you went over that huge bump. When I awoke in midair after being flung off the mattress, daylight flooded the truck storage area when the U-Haul's rolling door went whizzing to the ceiling. Now it's your turn—I paid my dues to give you guys extra space."

Bob can barely finish because Dan is laughing hysterically. Dan manages to stammer, "Hell no, I'm not riding in there. I didn't make you go there, that was your decision." Dan smiles to himself. *With Bob and Mom in the front, who knows what will happen—Bob might even let Mom drive.*

CHAPTER 16

Licensed

DAN HOLDS THE NEXT number tab in his hands. Sitting on the dingy cloth chairs at the Department of Motor Vehicles, we wait our turn. I'm in Oregon, utilizing my employer's generous parental care policy and trying to help my siblings with Mom.

Mom is rereading the *Oregon Driver Manual*. She has already taken the written test, unsuccessfully, numerous times in the last five months since she arrived in Oregon. This has become a source of tension and frustration for her and us; she wants to drive, yet we know it is not a good idea. She often asks about returning to New York where she is still licensed.

"Next," the woman yells, looking at the illuminated red sign to see which number to call out.

Mom, Dan, and I approach the counter.

"How can I help you?"

Dan says, motioning to Mom, "Maureen, my mom, needs an ID card. She hasn't passed the Oregon driving test."

The woman inspects all of us suspiciously. Dan towers over Mom and me, but speaks in a gentle voice. Mom is a 56-year-old, seemingly able woman. And I appear as if I'm eighteen.

Mom asks, "What are we doing here? Am I getting my license?"

I whisper, "We are getting an ID card because you haven't passed the written exam."

The woman behind the counter says, "I need to see your ID."

Mom dutifully slides her hands in her pockets searching for an ID, while Dan reaches in his pocket, retrieving Mom's New York driver's license from his wallet. He hands it to Mom, who then gives it to the clerk.

The clerk asks Mom, "Will you be retaking the exam at some point?"

"Of course I will. I'm studying so I will ace it." She proudly displays the manual, thumb clasped to the middle of the book, pages rolling inside the arch of her hand.

"There is no sense in getting an ID card if you will have your license soon. It costs extra money."

"That's okay, we would like to get an ID for the in-between time," Dan states diplomatically. This façade of independence we have created by not naming or addressing Mom's disability seems to be backfiring.

"In that case, I need to see proof of residence in Oregon."

Dan explains, "Mom lives with me, but all of her mail goes to our sister's house. However, we want my address on her ID." Technically, Mom lives in a double-wide trailer on the property adjacent to Dan. Dan, Jay, and Karen rotate spending nights at the trailer with Mom. During the day, she goes to an adult day-care center in Medford. Lyn, with a familiar Boston accent, has been hired to be "a buddy" to Mom. Lyn jokes, nudges, hugs, and easily redirects Mom. Karen receives Mom's mail, eliminating the possibility of Mom losing important bills or checks.

Again the skeptical clerk scrutinizes all of us. "Then a utility bill or bank statement?"

"No, there is nothing in her name that is delivered to my house."

Raising one eyebrow, she says, "Then we can't process your request." Ignoring Dan and me, the clerk deliberately slides Mom's license across the counter to her. Mom takes the ID.

"Do you want me to hold it for you so you don't lose it?" Dan asks, reaching for the plastic card.

Mom begins to pass the card to Dan. "Sure, that's a goo—"

The clerk motions Dan's hand away, saying to Mom, "Maureen, take responsibility for your own ID. Don't let anyone take your license away from you."

Every muscle in Dan's face tightens; he winces for a brief moment. I glare at the woman. Oblivious, Mom be-bops the card into her own pocket saying, "Don't worry, I won't."

Out in the parking lot, Mom reaches into her pocket. "Hey, here's my license; I'll drive."

"I'm driving today," Dan says. Shaking his head, his piercing eyes stare at me as he nods toward the DMV. Under his breath, he says, "That was a waste of time."

"Yeah, no kidding," I say, climbing into the back seat.

CHAPTER 17

The Escort

TWO MONTHS LATER, JAY and Dan stand beyond the airport security screening area. Mom's flight is called and pre-boarding begins. Mom is escorted by an attendant out of the waiting room. They have purchased this extra assistance as if for a child. The research doctors have requested that Mom spend three weeks at NIH to do extensive testing. When Mom first started participating in research, she said, "I want be part of research so you kids won't have to deal with this awful disease. That's my goal."

"There she goes," Jay says. "I need to use the bathroom."

Dan, Jay, and Karen have decided that having Mom live in the trailer is unsustainable. They do not have the time or energy to keep Mom occupied. Mom is continually obsessed and angry about not being able to drive.

A local foster home is expanding to add another resident and Mom is first on the waiting list. This trip to NIH will be the transition point. When Mom returns to Oregon, the foster home will be approved for the additional resident and the remodel will be complete. Mom will move directly into her new home.

Three minutes later, as Dan and Jay exit the restroom, they hear, "Hey, what are you guys doing?" It is a cheerful familiar voice.

Reeling around, Dan and Jay see Mom walking up to them. Dan asks, "Where did you come from?"

She points to the hallway that is marked "Do Not Enter. Arriving flights."

Jay interrogates, "I thought you got on the plane."

"I didn't know where I was going."

"We had someone walk you out."

"Well, I didn't know where to go. What are we going to do today?" Mom asks eagerly.

Dan responds, "We are going to get you on that plane."

Dan confronts the airline ticket counter employee. "Excuse me, the person who was supposed to 'escort' Mom onto the plane only pointed to the plane and told her to get on."

Jay interjects, "You must take her to the plane, put her on it, and help her find her seat and fasten her seatbelt. Make sure she stays on the plane until the doors are closed. She has Alzheimer's. She can't remember anything that you tell her."

The following day Dr. Eddie Watson, a NIH researcher, calls Karen. "Unfortunately, Maureen has progressed to the point where we cannot do any accurate cognitive testing. We will be finished doing all the physical tests on her tomorrow."

Karen gulps. "Tomorrow? We don't have anywhere for her to go. We are in the process of moving her into a foster home, and they will not have a room available until the end of the month." The trailer where Mom was living has already been offered to a family friend who is in the middle of a divorce and is caring for his 2 year-old boy.

Dr. Watson replies, "Because we requested her for such a long period of time, we will attempt to keep her here for a week while you figure out an alternative plan. Maureen's stay here depends on our ability to keep her occupied, as her emotions are tumultuous."

CHAPTER 18

Last Hurrah

DURING THE NEXT WEEK, my siblings in Oregon frantically jockey for openings in foster care homes. Jay moves the toys out of his kids' playroom to make room for a bed and dresser for "Grammie's" temporary room.

Mom has left NIH and is currently staying near Cape Cod with Bob, while our aunts and uncles keep her busy. I have made an emergency trip up from Kentucky, combining vacation time with parental care, to assist in this unexpected lack of coverage for Mom.

Mom and I have the cool gray evening to ourselves during our stay at Onset Bay in Massachusetts. I'm scheduled to be "on" with her, although I like to think of it as spending time together. It has been ten months since Dad's death.

After dinner, while it's still light, we walk to the deserted town beach to go for a swim. Mom has always loved the water and swimming. I sit on an old blanket on the sand, ten feet from the edge of the water, to write in my journal. The air is chilly, and I can't imagine going into the water now. Mom should be able to entertain herself, I think. She walks into the water, her floral swimsuit pulled tightly across her fair-skinned ballooning body. Lacking appetite control, she continues to gain Alzheimer's weight. I attribute this weight gain to her increasing desire for a taste of sweetness, one of her few remaining pleasures. She carries her mask and snorkel in her right hand. It has become harder for her to take a breath while doing the crawl stroke, so her caregiver, Lyn, bought her the snorkel. When the water reaches her upper thighs, I watch her dive, as she always has, headfirst into the water. "Brr, chilly," I mumble.

Wiping the salt water from her face, Mom looks at me and says, "It's beautiful—aren't you coming in?"

"I will be in soon," I respond, returning to writing. Mom swims parallel to shore for forty feet and upon stopping, looks at me.

"Kate, come in."

"I will be in soon," I repeat.

Recording the recent events with Mom, I scribble as fast as I can, pausing to glance up as she readjusts her snorkel and dives into the water, swimming out diagonal from shore. Sensing danger, I drop my spiral journal and my shorts as I hastily walk to the water's edge. Turning slightly with each stroke, she is heading straight into the bay.

I call after her, "MOM, MOM."

I jog into the water up to my waist. Mom is still swimming strong.

"MOM, MOM, stop for a minute. MOM!" I call, panic edging my voice.

I can barely breathe. *Is she doing this on purpose?* Is she trying to commit suicide? Or does she not have any clue? The cold air and water ratchet up my fear. I have been lifeguarding for five years, but never dreamed I would have to use my skills on the person who taught me how to swim. She's swimming strong now, but will she turn around? I race after her in a half crawl as I keep my head up to see her and call after her.

"MOM!"

I don't notice the water; I'm focused on her body and following her wake. I'm getting closer. We are way out. Ten feet from her, as if sensing my presence, she glances up and circles around while treading water.

Looking at me through her foggy mask, she spits out her snorkel and says excitedly, "You decided to come in after all."

I stammer, "Y...ye...yes, I decided to come in. Let's swim toward shore."

"Sure," Mom says with a smile. Setting the snorkel under her lips, we are off again, this time side by side. I watch her swim, chilled by her lack of fear and recognition of physical danger. Hearing a high-pitch whine under the water, I jerk up to see a boat driving by in the nearby channel. We are a long way outside of the swimming area buoys.

Upon returning to where we can touch the sandy bottom, Mom playfully starts a water fight and we swim one more lap together. An upper leg cramp grips Mom and she limps out of the water to rest. I help her with the towel as she sits on the blanket, getting out her *Reader's Digest*. Torn and well-thumbed, she has read this magazine many times but does not remember. Standing by the water's edge with a towel wrapped tightly around my shoulders, I scan the water, horizon, and sky. My heart is still beating wildly inside my shivering self-hug.

I think about Mom, her living will, and her right to die. She lacks control of her mind and thereby, everything. No longer allowed to drive, she is not able to take her life by crashing into a bridge structure in the way she attempted fifteen years ago when she was a pastor's wife and lacked control of her physical and economic situation.

During that time was when I first saw her cry. Dad was a Baptist pastor. Mom was taking care of a six-member family on a stringent thirty-dollar-a-week food budget. There were a number of days when her eyes and nose were red. I never saw the tears—only the evidence the tears left behind. Petrified at seeing my hold-it-all-together mother falling apart, I tiptoed around the house for weeks.

When she later told me about the attempt to take her life with a vehicle, she said, "God must have plans for me because I was accelerating toward the cement abutment at high speed. It would have been impossible to avoid. When I opened my eyes, I was driving down the middle of the road."

I never knew all the gory details; Mom and Dad kept them to themselves. But I do remember when our toilet seat at the parsonage broke. I was in fifth grade. Dad, without discretionary cash, requested extra money from the church to purchase a new one. A deacon thought it would suffice to give us his old crapper's butt rest; their family was buying a brand-new cushy seat with two inches of padding.

It was Grandpa Don, an elderly gentleman from the church, who brought the scenario to my attention. Sitting at the kitchen table one afternoon, I was eating a snack after my day of home-schooling. Mom was scrubbing the deacon's used toilet seat in the laundry room. Grandpa Don was making goulash with lots of hamburger—it was a rare treat for our family to have more than a mini portion of meat with a meal. He got out a big soup kettle, filled it with water, and set it on the burner.

Mom asked from the adjoining room, "What is that for? The goulash is already simmering."

He responded with a jolly wink and a shake of his cane, "Boiling that seat will be the best way to remove bacteria and germs." Then he grinned at me as he continued, "And it will also serve as the broth for the chicken soup we will give to the deacon's family as a thank you."

A seagull's squawk pierces through my thoughts; I turn to look at Mom on the sandy beach. She appears entranced by the small magazine that rests on her varicose-veined legs. Was she trying to take her life by swimming? Maybe it would be an easy and humane way to die, doing what she loves—swimming in the salt water on Cape Cod, her old stomping grounds, with her daughter to witness her last independent hurrah. Am I preventing her death? I can't imagine telling my siblings or her siblings that she died while I was with her. What would they say? It seems irresponsible. Maybe the bigger question is if I would ever forgive myself. I'm not sure I am ready to let her go, even if she is ready.

✳

CHAPTER 19

Poker Face

A MONTH LATER, MOM and I are sitting on a formal floral couch in the foster home living room in Ashland, Oregon. It is located on Normal Street, though there is nothing normal about it, with the multiple group homes and the various characters roaming the area. Veronica, with a wrinkled fair complexion and dainty features, is sitting in the corner near the TV. Earlier she showed me a photograph that was taken in her younger days when she was a model and in her words, "a real looker." Three other ladies sit in their favorite chairs. Julia, the owner and main caretaker, is preparing dinner and setting the table.

I've been at Julia's foster home since the early afternoon; it is my day and night "on" with Mom. This is her second day in the foster home and we, my siblings and I, are trying to help her settle into her new surroundings.

Distracted by Mom's decline and the continual strain on my siblings, I have moved to Oregon, leaving behind my environmental and social justice "dream" job in Kentucky. Only in retrospect do I realize that I wasn't meant for community organizing. I'm tender and have nothing of the thick skin or duck feathers required to "let everything roll off." I saw social bridges that could have been built—if only I had the energy, if only I hadn't been consumed by an avalanche that dropped me into a bitter freefall when my closest confidant, Dad, died. An avalanche in which I'm still being swept away as Mom's symptoms continue to increase.

Animal Planet is on TV, holding the attention of everyone but Mom and me. I hate TV and don't even own one. I pretend to be interested in the noise box, but feel like I'm wasting time. Mom actually likes TV, but today is uninterested in it. She is fidgety, going into her room and then returning to the couch near me. I flip through a home and garden magazine.

"What are we doing here?" she whispers to me.

"We will be spending the night here," I tell her.

"Come on, let's do something," she implores.

"We are. We're watching TV."

"I don't want to watch TV," she says.

"Well, I'm going to watch TV. You are welcome to find something to do yourself." We want this to work for Mom to be here at Julia's, but know it won't if Julia has to keep Mom entertained. My role is to help her get accustomed to the foster home, but not to engage her, letting Julia and Mom learn to work together.

Suddenly, Mom says piercingly, "I don't want to live with these old women."

I cringe; it is loud enough for everyone to hear.

"Mom, we can go to your room or out back to talk about this, but it is disrespectful to talk about it here," I firmly scold with furrowed brows.

Going outside to the patio, Mom begins to whimper, "I don't want to stay here. I don't need to stay with these old ladies. They are not even from my generation."

She is right; these ladies have twenty-five extra years of wrinkles, frail bones, weak muscles, and weathered spirits. I tell her, "You need to live with other people because you have Alzheimer's."

"I will go home," she says, "I'm leaving."

She turns her back on me and stomps beyond the white wood lattice and green ivy. I watch her thick body bustle away. I don't know if I should follow her or stay put. Torn, I slink to the corner of the house to see she has reached the beginning of the gravel driveway. Her body slows as she begins to turn around toward me. I dash back to the cement patio, not wanting her to know I was following.

A few moments later, she walks towards me briskly. With her right pointer finger in the air she declares loud enough for the whole neighborhood to hear, "This is BULLSHIT. I'm not staying here."

Silently, I pray for wisdom and guidance. My arms are folded across my chest. Chills from the cool air are compounded with fear. I feel tense, somehow responsible for the outburst and unable to stop it. *What happens when I can't make the world better, and it feels totally unfair, and Mom is losing control of her life in all ways?* I'm as scared as she is. I don't say anything. I don't know what to say.

Mom stomps off again, and I strain to listen for her indiscernible footsteps. I want to scream, *Mom, fucking look on the bright side of life! We are busting our butts for you and no matter what, you are never happy.*

She is gone longer this time. *Where is she? She will come back, won't she?* It is a gamble and I have never seen these cards before. I hold a poker face.

When she returns, I try to ignore the charade with a "tough love" approach. I pretend to be fascinated with the blue forget-me-nots in a glazed ceramic pot. "Look at these, Mom."

Distraction doesn't work today as Mom states matter-of-fact-ly, "I don't belong with all these old ladies. I'm not old."

She leaves again and this third time, I am humbled. I can't calm her down no matter what I do. *Can I be okay with her anger? She has a right to be angry and then some.* I wonder if she is ever coming back. As I stand up to look for Mom, her sneakers touch the patio edge.

Weeping violently, she is unable to stand up straight. She is bent over with her hands on her knees, looking at me sideways. White hair flops to one side as teardrops run off her red, chubby cheeks, staining the cement blocks underneath her. She asks, "Will you take me home?"

I don't answer. *What the hell am I supposed to do?*

She says, "You won't, will you?" Her words cut to my very core. "Why won't you take me home?"

Bam ... Mom has hit my button. *What does it mean to be family if I can't honor a desperate request?* When I was growing up, Mom and Dad had a policy that I could call day or night and they would pick me up if I was uncomfortable. It didn't matter where I was or even if I had been drinking. Now, here is Mom asking for the same and I can't reciprocate. Squinting, I fight the tears.

She is at the point where anger and despairing sadness meet. Dad's hug flashes into my mind and I remember the plaque that hung in the hallway: *People need loving the most when they deserve it the least.*

Counter to common sense, I ask her in a timid voice, "May I hold you?" knowing full well I may get clocked with her brute strength.

"Yeah," she says halfheartedly.

My arms are trembling as I wrap them around her tight, clenched body. Her chest is heaving as she sucks in air between sobs. I whisper, "I love you."

Slowly, I feel her arms come away from her sides and barely

touch me in a wimpy hug. I keep holding and breathing. "I'm with you and I love you."

"I love you too," she says as she hugs me tighter. "I don't want to stay, Katie."

"Mom, I know, but last night went really well. Dan stayed with you and you had a great night. I will be with you tonight," I explain for the sixth time.

"Okay, I will try it tonight. Tonight, and then that's it, right? We will leave then? I can't do this anymore."

"We'll see how it goes and talk about that tomorrow."

Walking back into the living room, Veronica notices Mom's demeanor and asks, "Are you okay?" She holds her brown cane and attempts to push her thin, feeble body off the upright chair.

Mom answers, "Yeah."

As Mom moves toward the bedroom, Veronica clutches Mom's arm and says, "Don't trust anyone—they are all out to get you." Mom stops, like a bodybuilder tolerating a 3-year-old hanging on her arm.

"Don't trust her," Veronica says pointing at Julia in the kitchen. "She lies and all the things going on around here, you wouldn't believe."

Veronica keeps talking as long as Mom is listening and Mom listens as long as Veronica talks. The other residents seem irritated and are shifting in their seats, and one nicknamed "Grandma" yells out that she can't hear the TV.

Julia's blonde hair floats away from her face as she walks into the room. She is wearing baggy denim overalls and a snug shirt that accentuates her fit, athletic body. She looks at me, and then she raises one eyebrow toward Mom and does a sharp nod toward the bedroom. Julia turns up the TV and talks peacefully to the residents. Veronica grabs her cane and jabs it in Julia's direction. I take Mom's arm, directing her to the bedroom, asking, "Do you want to read a book?"

Inside Mom's bedroom I say, "Remember, Veronica's medication is not right, so she is sick and often afraid. Julia is taking good care of her." Mom listens intently to what I'm saying.

When Mom uses the bathroom, I take the opportunity to check in with Julia. Julia says that she is working with Veronica's family and doctors to get Veronica's medicine stable, but so far, it hasn't worked. Veronica has been aggressive. Trying to quiet and smooth out the energy of the home, Julia is not sure it will work with Mom and Veronica, but says she isn't giving up yet.

Tucking Mom into bed, I read her stories from *Tales of the Kingdom.* I skip anything scary so it doesn't stir up any more fears. Mom interrupts me. "Your hair is beautiful."

Taken by surprise, I say, "Thank you."

"I'm glad you're here, because I like being with you," she says peacefully, as her heavy, swollen eyelids close.

Tension melts from my body and I relax into the bed. Setting down the large hardcover book, I play with her satiny white hair and think about the day.

Mom begins snoring, and I carefully move off the queen bed and slither into my sleeping bag, exhausted.

CHAPTER 20

✳

Smashing Vinyl

"WHY CAN'T I DRIVE?" These first words blister out of Mom's thin-lipped mouth as I pick her up at "work." It is commonly known as an adult day center, but Mom's overestimation of her ability yields its real name intolerable. *I wonder how many other 25-year-olds are picking up their parent from day care,* I think. *Is this really my life?*

"The doctor said you can't drive because you have Alzheimer's," I explain softly.

Mom's face is flushed and her right hand grips the door. "Why? Why won't he let me drive?" she asks, pressing her lips even tighter together in defiance.

Trying not to play into the unending fight dialogue, I take a deep breath and then say, "I'm sorry it is hard for you." Stealing a stealthy glance at her, I pull onto Route 5 on our way to Ashland. She is crying, but without tears. Her face is blotchy and contorted.

"Well, what good am I?" she demands. "Why don't I kill myself?"

I drive silently. Seconds tick by. Finally I ask, "Do you really want to kill yourself?"

"No, I don't want to," she states, barely audible, and then louder, says, "but if I can't drive, what good am I?"

"I love you, Mom. I'm sorry."

Abruptly, she concludes, "I'm going to New York. I'm going to get my car and drive back there. Let me off here," she points to the breakdown lane on the side of the interstate. Then, with an open upturned hand sweeping across the air in front of her, she says, "Let me off anywhere. I'm just gonna kill myself." Smashing the brown vinyl dashboard with her closed fist, she yells, "If I had a gun, I would do it right now."

I gulp; I have heard the stories from my siblings, but this is the first time I have had to deal with her anger. The white dotted line on the left of the car and the white solid line on the right join together in the hazy distance between my fingers clenched white around the steering wheel, trying to control both the car and this situation.

Again I repeat, "I love you. I would miss you if you died." In the back of my mind, I begin to wonder if what I'm saying is true.

CHAPTER 21

Broken Sunglasses

MEANDERING UNDER THE TOWERING Ponderosa Pines and California Black Oaks, Mom and I are on our way to feed the ducks. I attempt to slow down so that feeding the ducks will take a full ten minutes. It's another half hour before we meet Lyn; that is ten minutes with the ducks, ten minutes to the car, and ten minutes' driving time. It is Saturday, a year since Dad died.

Giving Mom quarters to buy corn from the candy-like dispensers, I watch as she fills her hand, walks to the edge of the cobblestone ledge, and dumps all the corn into the water without waiting for the ducks to swim across the small pond. Looking down at her hands, she slaps them together in an offbeat sideways clap.

"Well, that's done. What's next?" she asks, wiping her hands on her jacket, leaving behind dusty white prints.

"Don't you want to sit and watch them eat?" I ask, befuddled, then correct myself, saying, "I would like to sit and watch them."

"Oh," is all Mom says. She sits down next to me on the bench. A minute passes before she leans forward, twiddling her thumbs. "I'm ready to go." She takes off her sunglasses and begins to open and close them.

"Hmm," I murmur, trying to hide my annoyance.

Before our family recognized her inabilities as Alzheimer's, Mom's bread-making attempts vacillated between perfect plump, slightly sweet wheat bread and catastrophes of un-risen, doughy, or burnt bread. Dad would turn the disaster into a date to Sackets Harbor for an ice cream cone and to feed the ducks the inedible bread on the shore of Lake Ontario. I thought feeding the ducks would be pleasantly stored in her memory bank somewhere.

ChuBonk! Her sunglasses fall out of her hand onto the cement.

"Aw, ssshhit," Mom drawls.

Leaning down to pick them up, I see a big scratch through the center of one of the five-dollar lenses. Using my shirt, I polish them before handing them to her.

"Mom, they aren't even broken," I say, pointing out the positive.

She buys it for a minute, returning them to rest on her nose.

We walk three steps toward the Abe Lincoln statue when she exclaims, "They are ruined!" whipping them off to stare at the lens. "We will have to get another pair," she states emphatically.

"Hmm," I stall. She has another pair at home. Not wanting to take her into a store with her firecracker emotions I say, "We are meeting Lyn in ten minutes. That isn't enough time to get another pair."

"THAT'S BULLSHIT," she screams, throwing her hands over her head and storming down the path.

Okay, stay calm, give her space and time. Talking is not helping the situation. Breathe, Kate, calm yourself.

Mom's brisk walk leads her under the watchful eyes of Abe Lincoln, out of Lithia Park, past the steps leading to the Shakespeare Festival complex, and straight to the garbage can. Muttering angrily, she hurls the sunglasses into the wrought iron can.

As she turns the corner toward the Ashland Bakery Café, I run to the can and lean over to extract the glasses. They fall apart in my hands; she must have twisted them, intentionally breaking them.

"Shit," I say to myself before returning them to rest beside the rotting apple core. I dash after her.

Around the corner in the building's shadow, I slide my sunglasses to the top of my head. Her nose tight to the window, Mom is looking at the pastries behind the counter.

Forcing a fresh, chipper "Hello, Mom," as if it is a new day, I walk to her side.

"Mmmm," she says, looking at the yummy treats.

"Which is your favorite?" I ask, already knowing she will choose a cinnamon roll.

"A sticky bun, of course," she says, nudging me forcefully with her elbow, throwing my body off balance. Stepping back to catch myself, I smile weakly at her. She looks at my grimace and then at the top of my head.

She brushes her hand over her hair and feels around her neck. "Where are my sunglasses?"

I pause before tentatively saying, "They had a scratch."

"Well, it can't be that bad. Let's see them."

"You broke them when you threw them away."

"Oh." She looks down at her toes, slack-jawed and ashamed. Then she looks up the street. Jaw clenched with renewed confidence, she insists, "Well, I need a new pair." Shoving her hands into her pockets, she pushes off her toes, rocking to her heels; back and forth she sways, awaiting my answer, teetering on the edge of playfulness and anger.

✳

Dan and Mom stop at the bagel shop, Key of C. Mom was angry when Dan picked her up from the foster home this morning. Attempting to change her mood, Dan suggests a hot chocolate before taking Mom to adult day care. Mom enters the café with him, but after two minutes she tires of waiting. Annoyed at Dan for taking so long, despite the obvious line in front of him, she stomps out when the next customer opens the door. Dan pays, gathers the drinks, and follows her.

Seeing Mom a block away, he begins tracking her. They walk about three blocks when suddenly Mom disappears. Dan hurries to the last place he saw her, but she is nowhere around.

I lost Mom; just like that, she is gone, he thinks to himself, rubbing his chin. He stands against the row of buildings, searching up and down the street. *She will show up eventually.* He gulps his coffee, intermittently biting the inside of his cheek. *There is no use for both of us wandering around; if I stay still, I have a better chance of finding her.*

A half hour later, there is still no sign of Mom. Taking his hat from his pocket, Dan pulls the hat down over his red ears. It is chilly and her hot chocolate is cooling off. He sips on it to stave off the bitter cold. *Well, this plan isn't working.* He begins to search the town, trying to spy her white hair and purple winter coat.

Duda, dutat, his cell phone begins ringing.

"Hello?"

Karen asks, "Isn't it your day to take Mom to her 'work'?"

"Yes," he says confidently, not wanting to worry her or admit he has lost Mom.

There is silence on the phone.

"Why do you ask?"

Karen says, "Two police officers dropped her off at my door."

"Oh," Dan says, breathing out in relief. "Phew, I was getting worried."

"Are you okay? What happened?"

"She stormed away, and I followed at a distance. Then she vanished. How did the police get her?"

Karen replies, "They said she walked up to them saying she was lost. They searched her last name and somehow found me."

"I'm freezing my ass off out here and she is riding around in a heated squad car; no wonder I couldn't find her. Sorry, Karen, I'll be right over and try this again."

"No hurry, it's fine. She's grabbing a Diet Pepsi from the fridge, making herself at home."

CHAPTER 22

Too Safe

Names omitted

AS I SLIP OFF my shoes upon entering Jay's house, the garlicky aroma of a pasta dinner lingers in the air. Jay's kids are in bed. Mom is also asleep by now at Julia's foster home.

Jay greets each of us siblings with a hug and welcomes us into his home. In turn, we greet each other upon arrival: eye contact, a full, solid embrace with one or two deep breaths, and then the slow release. All the siblings who live in Oregon and our significant others have arrived.

Following the inviting and bitter scent of coffee brewing, we walk on the amber wood floor to the kitchen. The conversation begins as we grab a cup of tea or coffee and find a seat in the living room. Tall, arched windows overlook the Rogue Valley and the town below.

Spooning sugar into a mug, the last person in the kitchen asks in a raised voice, "Should Mom still be allowed to use knives when she comes over for a family dinner?"

From the rocking chair, a person projects toward the kitchen, "I want to let her use knives. Is preventing her from cutting herself worth restricting her freedom even more?" With coffee in hand, the last sibling enters the living room and sits on the futon. In a toned-down voice, the person in the rocking chair continues, "It returns to the discussion of value of life versus a life of value. If I get Alzheimer's, I want to enjoy the highest quality of life and most independence possible; I don't want to be restricted because I might get hurt." A hand tightly grips the gray ceramic mug as forearm muscles flex.

"Fuck, after she turned on me with the big pizza knife last year, I definitely do not want her using knives. I don't feel safe," a person promptly expresses with arms crossed.

"Why? What happened?" This sibling leans forward and the wooden futon squeaks. Stillness settles on the room. All ears are waiting for the explanation of this little-known story.

"She was telling that story about when she and Dad were first married and Dad chased the drunk out of their pizza shop with the butcher knife. As she told it, she was smacking the blade on her hand, acting out Dad's role." The person telling the story dramatizes it by chopping a hand through the air. "Then, she cornered me in the kitchen. I had to tell her to put the knife down. She didn't mean any harm, but with her lack of coordination and forgetfulness, it was not a good situation."

Covering mouth with hand, a person gasps, "Huhg!"

"Yikes, what about redirecting her to wash lettuce or something less dangerous?" a person seated on the floor asks.

"I think it is okay if she uses knives with supervision," a voice begins strong, and then hesitates. "But on second thought, you can all trump me; I thought she should be able to drive long after you didn't think she was safe—until I followed her home the night she blew through three stop signs on Southern Oregon University's campus and was completely lost."

The subtle pitter-patter of footsteps is on the stairway. We all wait, listening as the footsteps also pause. "Papa?" a high-pitched child voice asks.

Jay jumps up to attend to his little one. "Don't wait for me. Go ahead and keep talking. You can fill me in later."

After Jay leaves the room, a person says, "Let's take a break."

Ten minutes later, we re-convene.

"You have been quiet," one person says to another, after everyone has returned to the living room. "Is there anything you want to talk about?"

"Last week was rough bringing Mom home from 'work.' She kept saying she wanted to die and was going to kill herself." The speaker is rapidly clicking a pen, forcing the ball point in and out.

"She has done that with me also, probably to all of us now."

Still clicking the pen, a person says, "Nothing seems to calm her. What's going on with the Ativan? I don't think it's doing a bit of good."

"I talked with her doctor. He said that it can trigger anger, aggression, and confusion in some patients." On the floor next to this sibling is a tote bag filled with Mom's medical records and copious notes.

"Let me get this straight," a sibling erupts, brashly entering this segment of the conversation. "We're giving Mom something for her anxiety that has side effects of increased anxiety?"

Glancing at a vibrating cell phone to see if the caller is Mom, the sibling with the medical file replies, "Yeah, we're stopping the Ativan and trying to find other options. We'll talk to the doctor tomorrow."

The person clicking the pen has resorted to doodling. "What if her anger has nothing to do with the medication and she really does want to die?"

Crossing one ankle over an opposite knee, a person rubs a chin. "That brings up an interesting point. In her clear mind would she want to live this way? Are we effectively keeping her too safe, eliminating all her possible methods of committing suicide?"

"What do you mean?" a curious but reserved voice questions, forcing the subject into even more light. Suicide is something we have all been thinking about, but thus far have not discussed in an open manner.

Readjusting the ankle on top of the knee, the strong voice replies, "Well, we have taken away her use of power tools, driving a car, taking her own medicine, and now maybe using knives. And in addition to all that, she is under constant supervision. If she really wants to die as she is telling us, and as I would want in her situation, should we enable her death with assisted suicide? She can't really do it herself; she is clumsy and forgetful now. Or should we follow through for her?"

In a strained and pensive tone, a person responds, "I know I wouldn't want to live like that, but I don't know if I could help her die. I don't think I would be able to live with myself. It would haunt me forever."

The steady heartbeat-like flicker of the glowing fire inside the river rock chimney captures our attention and silences our words. Acceleration of the neighborhood traffic is heard beyond the subdued hum of the gas fireplace.

Breaking the introspective hush that has taken over the living room, an individual near the fire utters, "I think in her clear moments, she knows she has Alzheimer's and understands her surroundings. When she comprehends the reality of her life, the pain she feels fuels her anger and sadness. Maybe that is when she most wants to die."

"I wouldn't want to be in her spot, either, if I get Alzheimer's," a sibling insists. "But I don't think it's worth going to jail over. Most people—anyone without familial Alzheimer's—would not think we were doing her a favor."

Another person asks, "At the very least, should we quit intervening on her own attempts, like when Katie stopped her from swimming straight out into the bay?"

From the other side of the room comes a muted comment. "I don't know; instinct takes over in the heat of the moment."

"Well, don't prevent her death on my account. I have been saying my goodbyes to her for years."

Three hours into the meeting, a sibling stands up on tiptoes with arms overhead, stretching. Upon sitting down again, this sibling's head turns side to side until the neck pops. Hating the sound, my shoulders come up to my ears in a turtle shiver.

A sibling tapping on a yellow legal pad says, "The situation at Julia's isn't working. We have to figure out what our other options are. Julia isn't able to leave the other residents and follow Mom when she storms down the street."

"Can we find another foster home?" asks a person, fiddling with an orange mug scripted with *Our God Reigns*, a leftover from Mom and Dad's kitchen.

"Karen has found a few other possibilities, but none look as good as Julia's. There is only one located way out in the country-side that could accommodate Mom's wandering tendencies. I will go look at the three best homes on Monday. If anyone wants to join me, I will be traveling up to Eagle Point."

Sipping the last drop of coffee, a person inquires, "Why are you going to visit the place in Eagle Point? It seems too far away."

Shuffling papers, the sibling with Mom's medical file replies, "There are lots of decisions that I can make about general care for Mom and the way Mom's situation impacts me. For the bigger choices, I need you all on board. I'm willing to work to see if there is a better place."

A person seated on the floor leans into the window sill. "We appreciate that you are willing to make so many of the daily deci-sions. You are doing a great job, and I wouldn't want that job in a

million years. You make it so we don't have to discuss every little
detail."

Nodding, but ignoring the compliment, the sibling continues, "If the foster homes don't work out, the other inevitable option is a locked facility. The best one is in Medford; it's the clean-
est, has the best setup and staff-to-patient ratio. The one that we
are considering in Ashland is much closer, but doesn't seem to be
as good for Mom's needs."

Crossing legs and adjusting posture, the person on the floor
says, "I'd rather drive farther and know she is in the best facility
and getting the best care when we're not there." This speaker picks
up a tan Matchbox car that blends into the dotted beige Berber
carpet. Holding the wheels between the thumb and forefingers of
one hand, the other hand twirls the car around on its axle.

"I'll visit her twice as much if she is here in Ashland. Medford
is too far away for me to drop in during my lunch hour." From
the futon, this sibling says, "She doesn't care about where she is
located, who is taking care of her, and if it is clean. I think she
would rather live closer and have us nearby."

Getting up and moving toward the fireplace, a person says,
"I do think she wants to see us, but, at the most, we will only be
there three hours a day. I want staff that will engage her and treat
her well."

Another person asks, "Are we making this decision based on
what we want or what is best for Mom—or are they the same?"

Sitting on the fireplace ledge, the person says, "I think Mom
should be safe. Beyond that, would we feel relaxed hanging out
all afternoon with Mom if the facility is smelly and dirty? The
one in Medford has a nice outside area, so we can get away and
have alone time with Mom while still being in the locked home."
Setting down a water glass on the coffee table, it clinks into a
nearby teacup.

"I hate the idea of Mom being drugged," a depressed tone emits into the heady conversation.

"Drugged?" a surprised voice asks as a chin jolts upright and eyes look around, scanning the familiar faces to see if everyone else knows about this. "What are you talking about? Why would she be drugged?"

"How else do you think they will be able to control her anger and keep her inside of their facility?"

"No kidding! I never thought of that. What will she be like?" The question flies from a person gnawing on a thumbnail.

"She will be completely subdued. She will not be as spunky or engaging. I don't know if she will even be able to recognize us."

Biting off the white crescent nail, a person replies, "That's intense."

"We don't have any other options," a practical interjection is heard. "We're all exhausted. There's no way we can keep doing what we've been doing for her. In the report that NIH gave us evaluating Mom's abilities, we're compensating for her daily tasks by ninety percent. We've been putting our lives on hold. I think we've given enough; it's time we return to our own lives."

Swallowing, this sibling continues, "She poured her life out to us and we've done the same. No one can say we didn't try everything or we didn't give enough. I don't want any of us to end up like Dad."

A motionless hush settles over the room, like an altar call at church. Eyes are downcast. *Are any of us close to dying from caregiver stress? Have we done all we can?*

A couple of minutes pass before the next voice speaks. "Hey everyone, it's close to midnight. I'm exhausted and need to get up before dawn. Can we cover the decisions that need to be made or are we done for the night?"

"Uuhh ... we can't be done yet, unless we set up another meeting. We haven't decided what we are going to do with Mom."

Abruptly someone sings out, "Take her to your house. Are the rest of us in agreement?"

Laughter breaks the tension and follows with a couple "Hear, hear's" and a few "Aye, aye's."

One stern "No way" is heard above the chorus of voices.

"Okay, it's agreed," the singing voice continues, "majority rules. Sorry, you will have to deal with her for awhile."

A sarcastic "Ha, ha" is the deadpan response, but a smile follows.

Urgently, a sibling replies, "Seriously, I don't want to have another meeting. We've already had two this week. Let's make decisions."

"Okay," another person recaps. "We all agree we're ready for a locked facility if our impression of the other three foster homes isn't good?"

"Yeah, that's our only choice," one person says, while the rest of us nod in agreement. "I want to take her to the ocean for one last weekend before she is heavily sedated. Anyone else want to go?" A couple of calendars are removed from coats and bags to begin planning dates.

"Are you crazy?" someone asks, bringing a couple of mugs to the kitchen. "Have fun with the bathroom breaks every five minutes."

The sibling grins, "I need to go for me. And I want the kids to have one more weekend with Grammie. I want them to remember her."

Determined to get some sleep, a sibling prompts, "Okay, other than the ocean, if there's anything else anyone wants to do with Mom before she goes into a locked facility, we should do it now, as the move will take place in the next three weeks."

People stretch and start to stand up.

"Before we leave, I want to clarify something," one person says, spreading arms wide to claim everyone's attention. "I don't want any of you to change your life for me if I get Alzheimer's. When I can't drive or be by myself, stick me in a home, visit if you want, but please go on with your own life. Don't waste your time having three meetings a week discussing my newest decline."

"Whatever," a sibling replies, "I will want to spend time with you and help you out if you ever need it, which I hope is never the case."

Determined, the individual continues, "But I'm telling you, I don't want you to do this same thing of giving up your life for me."

Another interjection is heard from the other side of the room. "I feel similar, only stronger. If I can't pass the DMV test, take me out and shoot me. Put me out of my misery—it's not as if my quality of life will somehow return." The deep, serious tone of this voice sends visible shivers up the spine of one person who is clutching a pen. "No, don't shoot me," the voice continues, "I don't want that to affect any of you. Bring me out in the wilderness without any gear. If I wander home, keep bringing me out there until I don't return. In a week or so you can send a search party."

Slightly lighthearted, another person muses, "If I'm diagnosed, when I begin to show symptoms of impairment and NIH no longer needs me for Alzheimer's research, I think I will go to the front lines of some sort of war or conflict and protest for peace. That way, my death will be on my own terms and for a good cause."

Nothing more is said. Putting on our coats, we file out the door into the frigid December starlight.

CHAPTER 23

✳

Apt to Bloody a Lip

BBBRRRING. A MECHANICAL BIRD chirp interrupts my dinner. I sit still, determined not to be disturbed unless it is important. I'm in Watertown, New York, staying with Jim for a couple of months, hoping he will join me in Oregon. He is coaching sports at the school where he is teaching. The call is probably for him. The answering machine clicks on. It isn't the words that alarm me—it is the serious tone of my brother's voice.

"Kate, call me when you get this message." I scramble for the phone and press the rubbery green "talk" button as fast as I'm able.

"Dan, don't hang up, I'm here. Dan?"

"Kate, can I skip the polite stuff and get down to business?"

"Uhh, yeah, go ahead." Hearing the stress in his pointed words, I'm apprehensive. My hands clench the beige cordless phone. I slowly slide down the door frame between the kitchen and hallway to sit on the yellowing tile floor.

"Mom has been arguing and hitting other residents, and even tried to strangle one of them today. The staff thought she would have done serious damage if they hadn't walked in while she had the resident in a choke hold."

"What!?" I ask in complete disbelief. The few bites of dinner that I consumed solidify in my belly. Mom has been at Chapford, a locked facility, for a month.

"Do you really want me to repeat it?"

"No, not really, uh … I don't understand. What is going on? What provoked it?"

"We don't know; someone must have aggravated her. Karen and I are working with her doctor to adjust her medication. She will be drugged up for awhile. Chapford has warned us that if this inappropriate behavior continues, Mom will not be allowed to stay. They can't guarantee the care facility is a securely locked unit for Mom, because she probably has the strength and ability to pull the door off the magnetic lock."

Dan continues, "We want to take Mom off vitamins and things that prolong her life. Her quality of life is diminished and we hope to have the disease progress faster from here on, rather than slower. We will only keep her on pills that she needs to be at peace."

"Are we giving up on her?" I ask.

"Even if science comes up with a cure now, I think she has so many Alzheimer's tangles that her mind could never be restored to the original condition. She would forever be stuck in this stage. That seems like a miserable existence. Why would we try to keep her with us when she is already gone and has been for awhile— out of her mind?"

I listen without saying a word.

"Kate, I told Chapford, in no uncertain terms, to up the meds, even if it means Mom will be snowed. I also instructed them to stop Exelon, the Alzheimer's medication, if the doctor thought it would help her move on to the next stage more quickly."

"You are right," I say. "I never imagined this would happen. Is the person Mom tried to strangle okay?"

"Yeah, the resident is fine, but the person's family isn't happy."

"Do you need me to come home?" I ask, looking around Jim's apartment.

"No, there's nothing you'd be able to do anyway. I've been on the phone all day—I'm sick of talking. Do you want to say anything else, or have any other questions?"

"Uh ... no." I say hesitantly. "Thanks for calling to tell me about it." Stress seeps out of the phone and shimmies up under my shoulder blades.

Brring ... Brrring .... My body tenses. Abruptly, I close the book I have been reading. It has been twelve days since Dan called. I move swiftly to the phone.

"Hello?" I ask tentatively.

"Katie? It's Jay." His words are timid.

"Hey, Jay, how are you?" I inquire, concerned, as I hear the angst in his voice.

"Not great. Mom is oppositional, irritable, and violent, even after the recent medication changes. She threw a chair, snapped the leg off an end table, and broke a picture. On Friday afternoon, she bloodied someone's lip. She was immediately moved from Chapford to a psychiatric unit at a local hospital."

I imagine the off-white-and-maroon elder home and wonder what picture she broke. *Aren't they screwed into the wall?*

Jay continues, "Another med change is obviously necessary, but her quality of life, from my perspective, seems inversely related to the amount of meds she takes. When heavily medicated, she is not a threat to anyone, but she also has slurred speech, trouble walking, difficulty recognizing me and the kids. However, when she still recognizes us and is able to push Jake and Grace on the swings, she is also much more apt to bloody a lip."

"How is she doing now?"

"Yesterday, Dan visited and read her books. I tried to visit, but she was in isolation because she had been aggressive. I watched her on the video surveillance."

"What had she done?" It is terrible to think people have to be kept away from my mom to be safe.

"An employee said that she kept crossing a line on the floor and entering the nurse's station. I tried to explain to the person on staff that she has Alzheimer's, meaning she is forgetful—she probably wasn't trying to be oppositional or insubordinate, but is simply unable to follow directions. But I felt that I shouldn't say much, as I wasn't there when the incident occurred."

"What was it like watching her?" I ask, half scared to find out, but like watching a horror movie, I feel compelled to know the ending.

"It was awful," Jay confirms. "Mom was in a locked room with only a bed and one sheet. She would bang on the door screaming, 'LET ME OUT' and go to the bed and fold the sheet nice and neat. Then, she returned to the door, hollering, only to return and make the bed with the sheet. Soon after, she pounded on the door again. Peering out of the safety-glassed window she yelled, 'LET ME OUT.'"

CHAPTER 24

Chemically Bound

IN THE ELEVATOR, ON the way to the psychiatric unit, I link elbows with Karen to calm my shakiness. This is my first time to see Mom since I returned to Oregon after visiting Jim. We must pass through a screening where we say our name and who we are visiting while mysterious cameras record our movements. Artificial, dusty light has replaced the brilliant, fresh sun. Two minutes pass and my vision adjusts before we are allowed inside. A staff member closes the door behind us, *Kkkkhh click*, locking us inside. My eyes dart nervously around as I see the array of patients. One man in a hospital gown looks disoriented as he walks in a semicircle and then paces the hall. A pregnant woman wanders past us in slippers, and I wonder how being in the ward will affect the baby.

Karen guides me to the seclusion rooms. A tall male nurse lets us view Mom on the monitor. I'm thankful to see her first before interacting; it is a transition for my already shocked soul. Mom sits on the bed, then gets up and walks around it, out of her open door and into a hallway that leads from her secluded room towards the nurses' station. A locked door keeps her from reaching the nurses' station. Next, she wanders back into her pale pink room. Straightening the covers on the bed, she sits down again, folding her hands in her lap as she looks around the room. Like a mouse stuck in a cage repeating actions, her face is blank.

Holy shit! My mom is crazy. I have watched the changes progress so slowly that I didn't realize how different she has become from the rest of society. I find myself staring at her on the monitor as if she is a complete stranger with bizarre behavior. *Ba-Boom, Ba-boom*, my chest thumps.

"She is doing better now," a staff member reports to us. "She is able to be out of the secluded room for longer periods of time." Mom is now on four medications to help with her mood and behavior: Zyprexa, Depakote, Benadryl, and Haldol. In addition, the staff uses an intramuscular injection of Inapsine, a tranquilizer, for agitation on an as-needed basis. She slapped a staff member, and at one point she had to be restrained. Her youthful strength required many of them to "get her to cooperate." This is one big complication associated with early-onset Alzheimer's that sets it apart from late-onset Alzheimer's. With late-onset, most patients are elderly individuals who are feeble, regardless of the depth of their wrath. Mom, on the other hand, is as strong and stubborn as a wild stallion. Therefore, Mom's faltering mind in an unusually resilient and burly physical body is often an unprecedented situation for any institution.

Maureen Preskenis's reputation is ringing through the local medical community. The bad news is it will be harder to place her if Chapford doesn't work out. The good news is her reputation has warranted a referral to the best Alzheimer's specialist in this area, Dr. Whyzesol, a referral that Karen has relentlessly but unsuccessfully tried to secure since Mom moved to Oregon. On the doctor's advice, we want to discontinue all possible medications, especially targeted Alzheimer's medications. We do not want her to plateau at this level, remaining in an aggressive state; we would rather she drop into a more progressed stage of the disease so she will no longer be a threat to other people.

Will Mom recognize me? The attendant disappears inside the isolation chamber to guide Mom out. I turn to Karen. "How are you doing?"

"There is a pit in my stomach. This is a hard place to have Mom be," Karen says, looking at me. Turning our gaze away from the monitor and toward the seclusion rooms, her hand brushes mine as we stand side by side. She holds my hand in a tight squeeze until Mom's stocky frame emerges.

Wobbly on her feet and shuffling, Mom staggers in the doorway—totally drugged. As she gives us hugs, pungent onion body odor wafts out from under her lifted arm. In a slow, hoarse voice that I don't recognize, Mom says, "I love you guys."

"We love you, Mom," Karen replies. "Let's sit down over here." Karen tenderly slides her arm under Mom's forearm to help support her weight and guides Mom toward the teal plastic chairs at the entrance to the cafeteria.

Taking apricot-rose body lotion from my bag, I begin to massage Mom's feet. Karen holds one of Mom's hands while she opens *Anam Cara* and begins reading out loud. Her tranquil voice lulls us. The nearby fish tank hums and gurgles as the fluorescent bulb illuminates the tropical fish. Air bubbles circulate to the top, disappearing as they merge with the surface.

Mom's flesh is like hard plastic with a dry scaly coating, as if all her muscles and tendons have solidified underneath her thickening tissue. She has gained even more weight since the last time I saw her two months ago. I pray, *Please help some of my love massage its way to her heart.*

A peaceful hour passes as Karen's hushed voice reads to us.

Suddenly, we are reminded of our location in the ward by a man and woman talking abrasively loud in the cafeteria. One is sitting on the table and the other sits awkwardly on the back of a chair, feet on the seat. Tattoos cover the woman. Her torn shirt slips off her shoulder, and the man flexes his arm muscles as he looks down to admire himself. "…They were scared of me because I didn't give a fuck."

One finishes a story as the other jumps in, "Damn right, when I get out of here …" I shudder as their angry consolations echo into the hall.

Mom stiffens, and her shoulders bulge upward as she settles further into the seat, bracing herself. I continue to massage her long toes and take a deep breath.

"This feels good," Mom says, nodding toward her feet.

"I'm glad," I whisper, not wanting to draw the attention of the angry residents.

"What's new?" she asks.

"I came home from New York to see you. Jim, my boyfriend, is considering moving out here. It is good to …" the pregnant woman wanders past, pushing her brown hair behind her ear, eavesdropping on our conversation. "Uh, I'm fine," I sum up, distracted by the continual disturbing scenes being displayed all around me. Mom's body remains clenched.

"The sing-a-long will begin in five minutes," a voice down the hall calls out. Residents shuffle in the direction of our escape route. I look at Karen, lowering my chin slightly and raising my brows. She shrugs and points toward me and then herself and gives a half nod toward the door. I nod in agreement. Mom doesn't pick up on our improvised sign language.

"It will be a long time before we are home," Mom says. Karen and I listen without responding. I don't know what to say; she doesn't have a physical home anymore. She has lived in four places since she left Adams, New York, fifteen months ago and, depending on her behavior, she is teetering on five. We have tried to give her the best situation for her level of functioning, but due to her rapid decline, we have continually been forced to move her.

"Mom, let's go listen to some music. A woman is going to play the guitar," Karen says as I put Mom's socks on her feet.

"Will she go home with us?" Mom asks as we pass the pregnant woman, who is still lingering nearby. Before we need to respond, Mom continues, "I would like that."

As we enter the community room where the music is playing, Mom urges, "Let's go home. I've got to help my dad make dinner."

"Let's listen to some music," I say, knowing we have to distract her for Karen and me to be able to leave. A few patients clap to the music. The man who was pacing earlier erratically claps his hands together.

"I don't want to be home alone," Mom says. I bite the inside of my lip.

We sing "Puff the Magic Dragon" and hum the words we don't know. I hate this setting—the locked hospital, all these unpredictable people around me; yet I enjoy feeling her body next to mine. Mom may be the most volatile person here, as she is the only one currently living in the seclusion rooms. I don't feel threatened by her, but do know she is dangerous to others. I hate leaving, and I hate staying.

She blankly stares straight ahead and announces in a loud voice, "I like the guitar. That woman is good. I don't like this music." I cringe, trying to keep her polite, even in this setting. "What a racket!" Mom mutters during the rock and roll tune, but hums along when oldies, folk music, or hymns are played.

Karen nods to me and then slips out into the hallway. I whisper in Mom's ear, so she won't notice as a nurse replaces Karen, "I love you, Mom. It is good to see you again."

The staff will be putting her into the desolate restricted area soon after we leave. My chest aches. I have to get out of here. Mom turns to the nurse and I make my getaway, reuniting with Karen outside of the elevators as the guitar strums in the background.

Two weeks ago, Mom was released from the psychiatric hospital, returned to Chapford and placed in a new unit with different residents and caregivers. The previous unit's families justifiably complained about Mom's aggression, thereby necessitating Mom's move. I've been dreading visiting her. I would rather dance, drink, travel, or be a workaholic and ignore this segment of my life.

Spring is peaking in the greening grass of the outdoor area of the locked facility. I lead Mom to the bench outside; she is wobbly and slow.

She seems fairly calm, but she is physically shaking, as if she has Parkinson's. A medicated smile is propped on her face, out of context with reality. Mom's body is curved and taut as if bungee-corded forward from her neck to her toes. Her head is at a forty-five-degree angle, forcing her view downward. When I sit on the cement walkway at her feet, she is able to look at me. However, she doesn't hold my gaze, just looks at me long enough so I know she recognizes me, but not quite long enough to share a new connection. She is different, rigid, reserved—the evidence of a drugged and broken spirit.

Mom breaks silence. "It's good things are the way they are."

I ask, "Why?"

She says, "So everything else can do as it should. So things can take their proper place to make room for other things."

✳

CHAPTER 25

Inside Out Birthday

WALKING TO THE CAR, Mom is in front of me. I'm pawing through her swimming bag to be sure we have all of her essentials. Stepping off the curb, Mom tries to open the door of a green Volkswagen. I redirect her to Dan's brown Honda. Five months have passed since Mom was released from the psychiatric ward at the hospital. Drugged up, at age 57, she has settled into Chapford.

Mom takes a step forward and peers into the car. She leans down and takes another step forward. Her upper body is entirely in the car with her feet planted on the pavement. Lifting one leg, she sets her right foot on the car floor. Then, losing her balance, she moves her foot out and places it on the ground. Turning around to me, she exhales in exasperation, seemingly annoyed.

"Try sitting down in the car," I suggest. With her back on the top of the door jamb, she attempts to bend at the waist. As her weight begins to carry her into the car, she panics and grabs the door frame, hoisting herself to standing.

"You need to sit your butt all the way down on the seat cushion," I say patiently.

Mom huffs, furrows her brows, and sticks her face into the car.

Not wanting to increase her agitation, I walk around to the driver's side. With her upper body in the vehicle, Mom watches as I climb slowly and deliberately into my seat, pretending it is the most natural thing in the world. She follows suit by turning around. Then she half squats and falls backwards into the car, causing the Accord to bounce on its shocks. Using her arms the way an elderly person would do, she lifts her legs and pulls them in one by one.

"Good, Mom, now grab the door handle, right there. No, over further. Yep, that is it. Jerk it toward you. Great," I say as the door shuts. "Okay, now put on your seatbelt."

Mom's blank stare shifts side to side, up to the dash, and then out the window.

"Can I help?" I ask.

"Yeah," Mom says.

I lean over her body and pull the seatbelt all the way out and click it in the plastic clasp. Then, releasing the extra slack, it slides neatly into the door frame. Mom seems relaxed as she looks out the window. Conversation is sparse.

It is the middle of July, Mom's birthday, and I have arranged to celebrate it with her by bringing her on a special outing. Playing in water is something she loves but soon will be unable to do, as she is losing her physical abilities. I'm bringing Mom separately from Jay's family, who will be joining us; this way I will be able to leave on a moment's notice if she has a meltdown.

What am I doing? She can barely get in the car.

Driving into the parking lot at Emigrant Lake, I stop near Jay's navy Sidekick with teal and pink stripes.

"Look, Jay's here," she says, excited, and then asks, "Where is Jay?"

"He is at the waterslide waiting for us."

"But the car is here. Jay. Where is he?"

"We are going to see him at the waterslide."

Putting on our suits, the pace is slower than I'm accustomed to. I help Mom put in each leg and pull it up. She has gained so much weight in the past few years that I'm embarrassed for her, but she doesn't notice or think twice about openly changing in the dressing room. I ask her to use the bathroom before we enter the water, as she used to ask me. I have heard of her frequent accidents.

Mom's face lights up upon seeing Jay, Lori, Grace, and Jake. We all begin our walk up the path to the slides. Mom, stooped from her medications, trudges hesitantly. She cocks her head to the side to look up. Jake, age 2 ½ and Grace, age 4, are skipping and running ahead, but come whenever they are asked. They seem to know it is a big deal to have Grammie on the waterslides.

The huge stairway to the top of the waterslide is made of concrete and steel. We step aside often as other patrons run past. I hold on to Mom's hand and feel a smidge nervous. *Should I be behind her? Will she fall backward?*

Mom has always loved the water and anything fast or energizing. At the top, a lifeguard directs us to the two slides. We have to wait for the riders in front of us. Once we are up to the slide, he motions to us to sit down. Mom's bent frame steps gingerly into the small pool of fast-flowing water at the top of the slide. She is the oldest rider.

"Sit down, Mom," I yell from the slide on the right, with Jake on my lap. Awkwardly, she sits.

We have pink punch cards attached to our wrists that the lifeguard is supposed to mark. Baffled by the bizarre behavior—Mom's obvious mental impairment—he stutters while turning away without using his hole punch, and waves us on in bewilderment.

I start to push off to beat her to the bottom. I barely catch

myself with the pads of my fingers as she stands up when the cold
water surprises her body. Jake and I pause in the other slide. I sit
sideways, waiting, not sure Mom will take the plunge. I don't know
how we will walk down the stairs if she doesn't ride to the bottom.

Jay and Grace were waiting for their turn. Jay, biting on his
curled tongue that sticks out the side of his mouth, releases Grace's
hand and takes three quick steps forward. Fast and smooth, he
helps Mom to a sitting position with a motion that almost looks
like a tackle without the impact. Giving her a push down the
slide, he calls after her, "There you go, Mom." Mom shoots down
the slide without a word.

I push off extra hard. Jake and I laugh all the way down, but
I'm also trying to beat Mom. I don't know if she will remember
how to swim or how she will do on the slide.

Splashing into the water, I hold Jake and lift him to my waist
as we turn to see Grammie coming around the corner of the slide.
She has a radiant smile that pushes up her round cheeks. Seated
with hands on her thighs, Mom's azure eyes shine in the misty
water as she is dumped into the wading pool.

"That was great!" Mom exclaims. "Fun." My muscles relax as
relief sweeps over me. She swims out slowly, wanting to stay in
the water rather than walk in the chilly air.

Next, Grace and Jay rocket out of the slide and see the smile
blooming on Mom's face. Pictures are snapped to capture her de-
light.

Reaching the top of the slide for our second ride, Mom sees
how high we are and says, "No way. I'm not going down there."

"You loved it," Jay reminds her.

"Well, maybe I'll try it."

This time when she attempts to sit, Jay helps position her feet
straight in front of her. Then she bends a leg, putting the sole of
her right foot on the slide. Before she has a chance to stand up, Jay

immediately pushes her down the slide without waiting for the attendant's permission. As she rounds the first bend in the loop, a toothy childish grin is again plastered on her middle-aged face.

We stop to eat lunch. Mom has a few bites of her sandwich and drinks her soda. Ready for the next activity within minutes of eating, she begins to wander around. We clean up the half-eaten lunch. I take my sandwich for later and walk to the changing room.

Mom gets half undressed and grips a towel around her body. I begin to help her and she says, "You can't make me do that. I won't do that. I won't allow it."

Seeing her agitation, I change into my dry outfit and try to encourage her to change. She continues talking loudly and aggressively.

"Mom, I'm not trying to make you do anything. I'm helping you get dressed," I tell her in a calm voice.

"I'm not going your way. You can't make me. I'm not playing." Mom's voice is a notch below yelling. She is firm, but terror is evident in her voice. I'm afraid if people hear they will think I'm hurting her. She isn't talking so much to me as to herself.

I display all of her clothes on the bench and walk into the adjacent changing room to give her space. She must be reliving childhood abuse. I know she was abused, but I don't know the details. *Is this too much stimulus? Am I selfish to take Mom to do what I thought she would enjoy in celebration of her birthday? Something she will never do again? Could I have predicted that her response would change in an instant and the whole trip would feel miserable?*

I hear Jay's family from outside the wooded partition asking, "Are you okay?"

I walk out into the dazzling sunlight to talk with them. "We're fine. Mom's not cooperating and doesn't want to get dressed. I think she's remembering abuse from her childhood years. I'll stay with her, but it'll take some time. There's nothing you can do. Go ahead and leave if you want."

When I reenter the dim, wet dressing room, I sit down, put my stuff in a bag, and begin to brush out my hair. I don't talk to Mom. She is still fiddling with clothes. She has managed to put on her bra and underwear. Her big, white Hanes briefs are on inside out, but I'm lucky that they are on at all. After a few minutes, she looks at me. She has tried putting on her shirt, but it has become tangled and has fallen to the floor. Her face is a blank slate with no sign of emotional trauma.

I hold her gaze and then pick up her navy t-shirt. As I straighten the material and shake off the grit from the locker room floor, I ask, "May I help you put this over your head?" She nods. I pull it over her shaggy, damp white hair, put her arms in the sleeves, and help her slip it over her bra.

Her slumped stature has her staring at the drawstring denim shorts on the bench. She gestures towards them, so I reach for her shorts and motion for her to sit down. I put in a leg at a time. Before I have her stand to pull them the rest of the way up, I slip the blue sailboat flip-flops that she calls go-aheads onto her feet.

Finally dressed, I ask, "Do you need to use the bathroom?" She gives me a grimace of annoyance. Before she says anything, I add, "I'm going to the bathroom and leaving my bag on this bench." I set down my stuff and she copies, and then I enter a stall and she goes into the one next door.

At the car, I open her door and, not wanting to repeat this morning, quickly walk over to my side and get in. She gets in, but doesn't reach for the door, so I get out, hand her the shiny seatbelt buckle, and shut her door. Then, I climb again into the driver's side and lean over to help her with the seatbelt. She has her index finger through the square hole of the silver clasp. I help her remove the buckle from her finger and pull the seatbelt around her body and click it into the lock.

Mom is squinting severely. "My sunglasses, I need them." I rummage through her bag and pull out her old-lady, wraparound, black plastic sunglasses.

"Do you have a headache?" I ask, seeing the crinkle line in her forehead.

"No," she says.

We drive in silence to Chapford. I hang up her wet clothes on the towel rack in her bathroom and attempt to settle her into the scene of the locked facility. Walking like a gang leader scanning her neighborhood, she struts toward the activity room where people are playing with a ball. Despite her curved spine, she has better mobility than the other residents. She hovers outside the activity room, scowling at the excessive noise and activity.

"How was your day with your daughter?" one staff member asks.

Mom's gaze snaps from the activity room to the person in front of her. "I loved it. Was good."

"You're lucky to have a daughter who'll take you to a waterslide," the staff member says, surprised that I attempted it with someone who has Alzheimer's.

"How was it?" she asks, turning to me.

"Mom enjoyed it, but it was a lot of work," I answer. "I'll be leaving shortly," I say so she will know to keep Mom occupied. The caregiver smiles knowingly and nods.

Leaving the facility, I feel completely drained. Slumped forward on the steering wheel, tears soak my face. I whisper to myself, "Happy birthday, Mom. I love you. I'm sorry." I wonder if I stirred up emotion and created a ticking time bomb by not accurately reading Mom's abilities before this field trip, thereby forcing her out of her comfort zone. A time bomb the caregivers will have to deal with later. *Will Mom kick or punch anything or anyone today? Will she remember the fun she had on the slide?*

CHAPTER 26

✳

Dirty Old Man

THE DAYS HAVE AN Indian summer feel—bright and hazy after a chilly, windy spell, and the temperature is holding at a succulent ninety degrees.

Wearing my faded indigo shorts, a sexy backless tank top, and flip-flops, I enter the secret code to unlock the heavy maroon door that keeps Mom and the other residents inside. As soon as I enter, I see Mom seated in the dining room to the left of the door. She is at the end of the first table eating ice cream.

"Do you want some?" she offers me her precious dessert. She has been losing weight lately. Her face has new dry spots on it, and her flesh is bumpy.

"No thanks." It seemed appetizing from afar, but my stomach turns seeing the food and bits of pink medicine that remain around her mouth and between her teeth. I sit down next to her at the large wooden table. Mom is wearing a pair of baggy, elastic-waist blue jeans with a t-shirt.

Last month when I visited, I didn't recognize her. It was dinner time and I searched around the dining hall but she wasn't there, so I went to her room but it was empty. I found a staff person, who directed me to her table. There she was, halfway down the length of the table with her back to me. Her hair was rumpled and dirty. She was slumped over, sleeping and drooling. Drugged, she blended in with the other residents.

Mom is not as sedated today. She asks for more vanilla ice cream. There is one staff person who has taken a liking to her and has even brought in a Diet Pepsi for her from the outside world. This woman cheerfully gets Mom more dessert. Mom has eaten half of it when an old man enters the room. He is surveying the room with one eye. The other eye is squinted and shut tight. His opened eye lands on me. I notice his ugly bare feet and rumpled trousers, but try to ignore him.

Hunched, with crazed white hair, he moves toward us, saying, "You look pretty good," in a dirty, slimy, and intimidating growl. The evil tone of his voice and piercing leer raises goose bumps on my arms. Slowly, I let down my long blonde hair from a ponytail, covering up some of my exposed skin.

Awkwardly, I freeze, yet anger is burning inside of me. I bite down, scanning my options. This isn't my territory; I don't know the code of conduct or how to deal with this situation. Out in public, I would stare him down, walk away, or tell him to leave me alone. In this institution, he is sick and I'm the healthy one.

Still seated, I search the room for staff. There are none. One resident is mesmerized by the TV, another is nodding and talking to herself, and this new person is fidgeting with his clothes. Suddenly, I'm a minority in a mad house of individuals who are wandering, mumbling, and drooling.

Staring, he walks, haunted, around the corner of the table toward us.

Screeeeecch. Mom slides her chair back, blocking his path temporarily. She is standing at my left arm.

"Let's get out of here," she insists abruptly, leaving her second helping half eaten.

I mutter "Okay," while utilizing my peripheral vision to deliver fiery glares, but I don't move.

The hunched predator shuffles behind Mom, shoving her chair out of the way. Mom moves slow, seemingly methodical, blocking his view of me. Chills spill across my bare flesh in the sweltering heat as he walks behind us.

Mom, determined, concerned, and in complete control, leans toward me. "Are you okay?"

"Yeah," I say, but I'm not convinced. I can still feel him.

Then, to my amazement, in the precious seconds during which Mom blocked his view, the stalking man vanishes and, like a boy exploring a new world, he fixates on the next item of interest: the shiny gold door handle.

Mom grabs her chair with one arm and pulls it up next to mine. Clasping my forearm firmly she asks again, "Are you okay?" Her mouth hangs open, waiting for my response.

"Yeah, I'm fine. Thank you." Mom believes me this time.

I ask her, "Are you okay?"

"Yes," followed by "*ffftt,*" as she sucks saliva back through her lips before it slides completely out of her mouth.

✳

CHAPTER 27

Mords Wixed

A WEEK LATER, I visit Mom again. I'm wearing jeans and a long-sleeve shirt. "Mom, let's go outside." I lead her to the garden walkway that is secured inside a fence eight feet high. She shuffles and scuffs her feet as she walks. We sit on our usual bench. Asking her permission, I push record on my mini tape player.

Then, I get my apricot-rose hand lotion out of my purple bag and ask, "May I give you a foot massage?"

"Oh, sure, that sounds wonderful."

Taking off her cotton sock, I separate her toes to remove the fuzz balls and examine her yellowing toenails. It is my secret way of connecting with her. I can't stand to talk with her all the time, as the conversation goes in circles or nowhere at all. When I touch her, we connect without words. Crouched on the ground, I'm able to see her face without effort. Her shoulder muscles have become hardened lumps, forcing her to slouch.

"Mom, are you afraid of dying?"

"No, I'm not afraid of Diane," she responds. Then, a quick frown hits her cheeks, followed by a slight smile as she shrugs, lets out a sigh and says, "Ppppfffff …. That got changed."

"You mean dying?" I ask, trying to help her.

"Yeah, I'm not afraid."

Sitting peacefully, I work the tight muscles in her calves all the way into her ankle bones. Her flesh is like an unopened tube of toothpaste—I massage the surface, knowing it is doughy inside, but the contents are packed full with no place to release. Mom is taking in the massage, one of the few moments in her life that she isn't fidgeting or wandering.

"Will you be my guardian angel?" I request.

"Yes, I will build anything for you," she responds. Mom remodeled our house in Adams by refinishing the wood floors, putting in bathrooms, adding electrical outlets and insulation, making curtains, and painting. I don't doubt her intentions or past abilities. If she didn't know how to do something, she would teach herself with an "I can do it" attitude.

"You don't have to build anything," I explain in case she doesn't understand. "I'm wondering if you will be my guardian angel," I repeat.

"Yes, of course I will," she states emphatically.

Replacing her socks and shoes, I move to rub her hands and arms. She tells me my fingers are purple. Is she able to see auras? As I rub her right upper arm, I feel a big bump in the fleshy underside near her armpit. It is new. There is no outward sign of trauma and she says it doesn't hurt.

Mom says, "Just being here ... sitting ... next to you ... is nice."

"I like it also." My voice shakes with emotion, thinking about who she used to be before getting Alzheimer's. I don't try to protect her from my tears. I let them come.

Mom immediately seems clear, initiates a hug, and tells me, "I love you so much. You are so precious."

Mom's glance catches something in the rich green grass. "Those flowers, the pink ones—" she nods, her voice stopping unexpectedly in mid sentence.

"Are beautiful?" I ask her, after an extended silence.

"Yes," Mom responds.

Barely visible in the deep lawn are the tiniest and most delicate pale pink flowers.

I ask, "Is it hard for you to not be able to say what you mean and have your words get confused?"

Mom says, "Usually, but not today. That didn't bother me."

"Jay's been here," Mom tells me.

I smile that Mom remembers a visit from one of us, and think fondly of Jay's sincere and playful nature. I remember the most recent conversation I had with him. He told me Mom has been weepy each time he has been visiting lately. She hasn't been weepy when I've seen her. I've been the one crying.

I ask her the meaning of life, thinking she may be getting the scoop from the other side. She says she doesn't know. She talks mostly gibberish and is physically quivering.

Touching her flesh, it vibrates under the surface, a buzz similar to static on a phone line. I ask, "Mom, you feel shaky to me— do you feel that on the inside as well?"

She looks me in the eye, which is a big thing now that she is hunched over, and with surprise says, "Yeah."

"Why do you think you are trembling?"

"I don't know," she responds as if thinking to herself. Taking a full breath, she exhales, resting her chin on her chest. I try to rest my chin on my chest, and quickly realize it's as uncomfortable as it looks.

"I will be going soon," I tell Mom, knowing I'm leaving in fifteen minutes. I hate departing without telling her, but sometimes I have to sneak out so she doesn't get angry or teary. I want some part of her subconscious mind to know I told her goodbye.

"Where?" she asks.

Thinking as fast as I can, I respond, "To come see you again," trying to hide that I will be gone in between, and not wanting to upset her.

"Good, I'm glad," she says.

CHAPTER 28

＊

Gazing Between Worlds

IN HER ENGAGEMENT PHOTOGRAPH, a black shawl drapes off Mom's beautiful bare girl shoulders. The purpose of the photograph, which hangs outside of her room, is to help Mom identify her room despite her receding memory. The photo has hung on a wall of our various homes ever since I can remember. I recognize her face, but not her clavicle line in this photograph. The clavicle I know has a sharp, heavy crease from her gouging bra strap. Her long, blonde silky hair is in a French twist, a far fetch from her current short, rumpled white mop. The old photo is torn from being moved, as Mom was forced to change rooms and buildings with her ongoing anger episodes.

Rank urine stench shoots to my nostrils, making my eyes water. I hold my breath and knock lightly while pushing the door open. "Mom?" I ask.

Immediately, the smell is worse—the ammonia of a windowless outhouse. There is no clean air to be consumed. I prop open the door with a wooden straight-backed chair.

Sitting on the edge of her bed Mom watches me enter and says, "Hi." Then, smiling, and with a lighter, more engaged tone, "Hi, Katie. How do you like the beach?" she asks.

She must be remembering my years of lifeguarding—the weather is right. Gasping for air, I move to the windows and open them, letting in the sunny, fresh oxygen.

"I love the beach, probably as much as you do," I respond. Then, I pretend to look outside as I press my nose to the screen, gasping for air. After I catch my breath, I search the rug for wet spots from a urine accident. Opening the bathroom door, the stench is overpowering. Liquid, most likely urine, is on the floor between the toilet and the shower. I assume Mom's roommate had an accident. I have only seen her in bed crying. She doesn't seem to have any social skills.

Meandering out into the community room, music and nail polish fumes fill the air. The activities director and residents are listening to the radio.

Bum bump bump bumdada da dada dadada … "These are a few of my favorite things," *The Sound of Music* song, familiar to Mom, touches our ears.

Stiff, seated bodies line the room. I gently take Mom's hands in mine and start dancing. I slide slowly, and she seems confused at first as I move sideways rather than forward or back. Then, she shuffles sideways herself, and, closing her eyes, she listens to the song. She is dancing with me and a smile spreads across her face. We finish the dance and continue our walk.

Mom says, "That helped."

I ask, "Do you like dancing?" I remember spontaneously dancing with Mom in our kitchen when I was in high school.

"Yes, but I didn't know I could do it," she says.

My chakra right in the middle of my chest is fluttering—not in pain, but in an exciting, fun way. It feels as strong as a heartbeat but with a different rhythm.

❋

Later in the day, Mom is sitting in Chapford's living room in a dark, high-backed chair with gold dots in square patterns on it. She looks at a space in the middle of the room, and her gaze widens as if her eyes are focusing on the in-between space. I calculate the depth of her vision; the wall is too far away. The couch is too low and close to be where her eyes are concentrating. It is somewhere in the middle. Mom doesn't have a blank stare that comes over someone spacing out; it is active, as her pupils move, apparently following action.

"There's God." Mom says excitedly, almost to herself.

"You see God?" I ask. I try to look cross-eyed in the same space, to see if I may see God. Chills course up and down my relaxed arms. I anxiously wait for Mom's revelation, but don't want to disturb it.

"ZZZZ-mazing!" she exclaims, nearly breathless, vivid with anticipation.

She continues, "I'll be with her soon." I freeze all voluntary movement, wondering what that means, and I'm pleased that God is female. I used to joke about it with Dad, but Mom now confirms it.

I mouse whisper, "How soon?" leaning toward her ear, but still staring at all the blank spaces in the room.

"Don't know." Her trance-like voice is distant and flat. Her head tilts to the right and she continues, "Soon. I got to help someone first." Her tone is matter-of-fact, nearly emotionless. "Do some good," she adds.

"Mom, you help everyone." I wonder what her secret mission is.

During that month, Dan takes Mom out for a walk in the elementary school yard behind Chapford. They are on a dirt path around an open field. They walk in circles because Mom doesn't know the difference anyway, and it is easier than going on a long walk and dealing with a potential emotional meltdown. Ponderosa Pines divide the path from the nearby homes.

Mom motions to the middle of the field. "Who is that over there?"

Dan asks, "Over where?" There is no one in sight.

Mom says, "Over there."

Dan replies, "I don't see anyone, Mom."

"Oh, it's Dick, your father," she says with relief and then playfully jabs Dan in the ribs.

Dan says, "Err, aah, hi, Dad," in a passive voice, half in jest.

Mom takes him seriously. "No, he's not there," nodding to a few feet away, "he's over there." Mom is pointing to a grassy area thirty-five feet away.

Dan, smiling now, amusing himself, says, "Hi, Dad," in a much louder voice and with a wave of his hand. He can barely keep from laughing.

Mom seems content as they continue walking in silence. After ten minutes, they decide to rest on a wooden park bench. Dan puts an arm around her.

Mom peers again to the middle of the field and says, "Look! There they are, and there's Dick!"

Dan is surprised that Mom is gazing in the same place and seeing Dad again. With her faltering mind, she couldn't have held that idea without a reminder. Dan looks cautiously toward the field.

Mom goes on, "Sometimes when he can't personally be here, he leaves behind his angels to be with me."

CHAPTER 29

Endless Stutter

IT IS LATE SEPTEMBER; I'm at Chapford showing Mom the pictures that I had developed from her birthday at the waterslide park. I'm both excited to share them and nervous about how she will respond. All my life, she would eagerly engage over a family photograph; however, since the disease, predictability is nonexistent.

Taking the pictures out of my hands, she stutters, "Ddddd, dddd, dduduuddd, bbbbuuu," as she clumsily flips through them. It is her new way of communicating when she is excited about something, a nearly endless stutter with a big smile. "Mmwwa." Bringing the photograph to her face, she puckers her lips and kisses the floppy, colorful photo.

"It is the best picture I have ever seen. I was hommified," Mom continues without my prompting. She is holding the picture of Jay, Jake, Grace, and herself at the base of the waterslide. Putting it on top of her Alice blue jewelry box, she says, "I sat there and I sat there. I put too much on, I put too much on. It was that good.

"Oh, my word, I tried to tell someone this here, but nobody could say. I can't imagine this here. I can't smm—someone would say you couldn't do that. I could have walked off the edge and I have never done that."

"Mom, were you trying something new?" I ask.

"Yeah, I can't tell you how good it was," Mom answers.

✳

"Mom, you know they are making breakthroughs with the Alzheimer's research that you have been contributing to?" Today, the research doctors have notified us that through her specimens, they have located the Alzheimer's gene that is affecting our family. Mom and I are sitting on her bed. The familiar bedspread has splashes of brown, pink, and green on a white background. It has become stained in the last year, but Mom doesn't seem to notice or mind. It is something Mom would have scrubbed out or bleached to death two years ago.

"I want 'em, they better get a keep 'em." Mom is insistent as she nods vigorously, her emblazoned eyes speaking louder than her words.

"All the times you have given blood are paying off," I tell Mom, wondering if she really understands. I remember she used to say she would do anything it took to prevent her children from getting this terrible disease. This is a step in that direction.

"Oh, that's fumous," She says. Sighing with relief, she settles into the bed as if in deep thought.

"It's great, huh?" I ask, smiling at her choice of "words."

Mom is still for a few moments before scrambling to a standing position with dramatic flair. Breathless, she exclaims, "Ha— they. Ha—. They did it for me. Oh, ah, it's so beautiful." Giving me a firm exuberant squeeze, she squishes all the air out of me.

CHAPTER 30

Greedy Genes

Names omitted, researcher transcription

FORTY MEMBERS OF MY extended family are seated in a semicircle around two research doctors, Dr. Albert Green and Dr. Eddie Watson. We are at Brigham and Women's Hospital in Boston. It has been a month since the researchers from NIH found the mutated gene that causes Alzheimer's disease in our family. They called this meeting to explain finding the gene, the impact this news could have on us, the opportunity to find out our genetic status, and the importance of our family participation in research. NIH provided plane tickets for my siblings and me to attend this meeting.

An energetic buzz hangs in the air like static electricity, sparking to life with any movement. A conference phone located in the middle of the room is linked directly to Dr. Lance Gregory of NIH, a superior of Dr. Watson. The shades are drawn to allow the three video cameras to fully capture this historic occasion for our family. Afraid to move, I'm glued to the chair. *What if I miss something important? And it all seems important.* I scrawl notes in an effort to get a handle on this huge announcement.

"What was special about your family was upfront right from

the beginning. 'We are concerned about ourselves, but we are also concerned about our children.'" Dr. Albert Green recalls his first interactions with our family. "And it was at that moment that I realized that this was a different story. This was not the typical one-to-one doctor-patient relationship, because the ramifications of what we have here affect future generations. It became clear the family members were not just interested in themselves or their children, but also had a broader goal: research, because it would benefit the wider community. Nowhere is this better exemplified than in the bike ride [the Memory Ride], which is an extraordinary gift to the Alzheimer community."

I glance at my uncles John and Eryc, who began the Memory Ride. Tired of feeling helpless in the face of this disease that is wiping out our family, they organized a bike ride to raise awareness and money specifically for Alzheimer's disease research. Butch, another uncle who has been active in the ride, is operating a video camera. In his late 40s, Butch recently developed early symptoms of Alzheimer's. Eerily, the disease continues to creep through our family. Fran, my aunt, is in a care facility—as is Mom.

Dr. Albert Green continues, "Agnes [my grandmother's twin sister] ... had her brain examined microscopically, and that has turned out to be an enormous gift to everyone in the family, and the reason for that is we, right now, would not know we are dealing with Alzheimer's."

"Right from the beginning we were looking for a gene ... the gene that can cause Alzheimer's disease in your family has one letter within that gene that has a mistake, which, when inherited, leads to Alzheimer's. When you get the DNA from someone's blood, you can find this deviation. So the very first thing we wanted to do when we met your family was to get blood, and look for one of those mistakes .... We made arrangements to get a sample.

"The reason we chose Fran was because at that time, we were

pretty sure that if anyone was going to have the deviation that was still living, it would be Fran. At that point, she already had clinical Alzheimer's disease; we weren't sure exactly that is what it was, but we had a very high suspicion—she had memory loss, she was already affected.

"… That blood sample was taken at UPC Daze Memorial Hospital by Dr. Sam Kline, and I made arrangements for that doctor to send the blood to a leading Alzheimer's researcher—a doctor who discovered one of these mutations, Dr. Geoff Smith.

"Dr. Smith did not find any of the known [already discovered] mutations in Fran. Now, we figured we couldn't find one of those three genes; we are going to hunt down the fourth gene. We are going to find all the family members who might be affected or might not, and begin the search for a fourth gene.

"Another very well-known researcher at the NIH, Dr. Phillip White, discovered the very gene where we found the mutation in your family. Dr. Eddie Watson was able to actually find the mutation—which is the subject here today.

"… But the question we have to answer is what went wrong? How did we have all these blood samples for almost four years and not get the mutation, and then find the mutation now? So, as soon as I heard about this, I called up Dr. Geoff Smith and asked, 'We have another sample down at NIH, and now there is a mutation. What happened?'

"The sample that Dr. Watson tested was from Maureen. Now, if this was a mutation in the family, both sisters should have the same mutation. It wouldn't make sense that one has it and one doesn't. So Dr. Smith tested not only the sample he got originally from The UPC Daze Memorial Hospital, but he also tested a different sample from Fran. And the sample from the UPC Daze Memorial Hospital was still negative, but the new sample on Fran now had the same mutation that Maureen has.

"So what happened? There are only one or two possibilities. The sample got mixed up at UPC Daze Memorial Hospital. It was either mislabeled, or drawn from the wrong patient, something happened there, because we now have been able to confirm that Fran clearly has the mutation—"

Quietly, almost meekly, a voice speaks from the side of the room. "The other one was mine," Bob says, his brown wide-brimmed hat casting a shadow over the smirk on his face.

Laughter erupts from people around him. The researchers have not disclosed our genetic status to individuals in our family, so we have no idea whose sample it really was. Then, louder, Bob continues. "I don't want to be greedy," he says, raising his hand, staking claim to a blood sample that is negative for Alzheimer's. His face has a full jolly smile. "The other one *was* mine."

As the laughter dies, my uncle's voice is heard. "Nice try, Bob."

Without hesitating, the researcher smiles at Bob, saying, "We will let you know about that." Then, his strained countenance returns. "So, this has been a setback, a three-year setback."

During our fifteen-minute break, I use the bathroom and then dart to a deserted hallway. I whisper into a digital voice recorder, trying to hit all the main points that will jog my memory later, as well as noting my emotions and thoughts. An uncle walks by me, clearly confused that it appears I'm talking to myself. He nods toward the meeting room. "Three minutes until we start again."

Now, I'm sitting in the same plastic chair munching on a cookie and sipping red punch. When others around me take their seats, Dr. Larson begins.

"Even though we can't say when, if you have the mutation, you'll get the disease, unless something else strikes first. And when

I say you will get the disease, nothing is a hundred percent in medicine, so I would say you're gonna get the disease with ninety-nine percent probability if you have the mutated gene. The probability is very, very, very high." Dr. Larson adjusts his glasses. "It is a serious, serious mutation. This conversation today is a big deal."

From the first row, an uncle asks, "Do you have any figures to the survival rates in life to age 50 or 60? What percentage of us would die by age of 50 or 60 from other causes?"

"... It is very different in different families ..." Dr. Larson gestures to his left in the direction of my aunt. "I was extremely sad to learn today about Kathi; ... Kathi has cancer. Cancer can strike anyone. Some people say there are even genetic predispositions for that."

Kathi is lying on the floor; her arm cradles her head. Rotating positions from sitting to lying down, she is seeking relief from her constant pain. Kathi's family has driven up from North Carolina for this meeting.

I put down my half-eaten cookie and slide my drink under the chair. My belly is churning the few sweet morsels into a violent storm.

Dr. Larson takes a sip of water and clears his throat. "Everybody now has another decision to make, and that decision has to be made around all the most significant things that people do, like get married and have children and even enter into relationships. Because when you know there's a possibility of the mutation, it is in your power now to decide if you want to be tested and who you will tell.

"We are now entering the waters of genetic counseling. Some people want it for their own personal planning now that planning has very grave implications. Some people mean planning like financial planning, thinking of their children. But, I am going to be very frank with everyone here, there are other people that when they are talking about planning, they are actually talking about suicide. There are studies—one occurred very recently in Sweden. They found a family with a mutation and they were informed, and a number of people in their family did take their own life. I think that because this is so serious, we need to know what the guidelines are for genetic counseling."

I gulp, seeing the grim ceramic faces that are also looking at me and at each other.

At least a half hour goes by, while my brain is lost in a twisted "choose-your-own-adventure" series. First: I have the gene, maybe I get married, maybe I have kids, I get sick. Next: I don't have the gene, maybe I get married, maybe I have kids, I take care of everyone else in my family who might get sick. I keep trying to pull my brain back into the room, but it is playing out possible scenarios. Next: I have the gene, I do research. Next: I don't have the gene, I get depressed I have wasted half of my life in fear of having the gene. Next: I move to Hawaii, I ignore the gene and Alzheimer's. Finally, I hear the research discussion again. I look at my illegible notes. Was I writing about my daydreams or was I still taking active notes?

Dr. Larson says, "There should be no compulsion on anyone's part to participate, here. I know many people in this family independent of the research, and in some ways I won't even know who is participating." He is a local researcher not associated with NIH.

"It is a lot of fun to have an eight-inch needle in your back," a person from the older generation murmurs.

"That was going to be my next question: is NIH planning to test our generation, more than blood tests?" a cousin asks.

Dr. Watson jokes, "Ahwaa, waa waa wa," offering an evil cackle, implying he enjoys torturing us with spinal taps.

Everyone is laughing.

Another cousin yells over the laughter, "I can tell my years of bugging him [Dr. Watson] to join the ride"—she is referring to the Memory Ride—"are coming back to haunt me."

One uncle asks, "Are you willing to stab them in the back?"

"Oh, absolutely," the researcher deadpans.

The serious question—whether research will include cognitive testing and spinal taps on my generation—is then directed to the white conference phone. Everyone leans in closer to hear as Dr. Gregory's voice responds, "Yes, the cutoff is eighteen for research, but anyone over eighteen who is willing is welcome. We would be doing more than a blood test. We would probably be doing brain imaging, blood tests, certainly cognitive testing, and offering a lumbar puncture—"

Scraping his chair loudly on the floor, an uncle stands up. He interrupts by shouting, "Ohhh, that is such a great awwhffer!"

"I thought you would like that," Dr. Gregory replies.

Dr. Watson picks up the conversation. "The power of the lumbar puncture is in studying the fluid. We can find indications and markers already known about the illness. Beta amyloid and tau are two proteins that are seen in a significant number of people with Alzheimer's disease. We are following to see what indicators predate your sickness. It is a bad time to be going to the doctor when your memory is already failing you.

"Now there are medicines that are geared toward the symptoms of memory loss—Aricept, Exelon, and Reminyl. But that is not enough. The drug companies, researchers, and others around the world are trying to develop interventions that get to the core of the illness.

"When you find a therapy that is geared toward slowing down the accumulation of beta amyloid, the plaques, and altering the inflammatory cascade that is caused by damage to neurons, these are therapies geared towards slowing the illness down at the core.

"The power of your family will be in contributing to information about these basic mechanisms, but also hopefully getting in line for some of these types of interventions."

Without premeditation, I realize my gaze is on Butch as he adjusts the video camera. Will Butch get an intervention? Will his past efforts to find research projects and raise money for research pay off for him? Suddenly, I feel guilty looking at him, as if I'm drawing attention to him. Discreetly, I take a sip of my juice and doodle in my notebook.

"How many of us do you need to make it worthwhile to do research on our family?" asks a cousin, propping elbows on knees.

"Twenty," Dr. Watson responds, without hesitation.

I quickly peek around the room again. *Who is able and willing to commit to being part of research? Do we have twenty?* I notice others are also counting, either with a tip of the head or a wiggle of fingers as they look from person to person, also trying to guess who is willing to be involved in research. A few family members keep their gazes down, obviously still weighing the situation.

"Is our parents' generation included in that twenty?" one of my siblings asks.

"Yes," Dr. Watson replies.

I relax a little. That gives us an extra nine people who have already participated. However, does that mean our parents' generation has to be involved in future research? Mom and Fran are too far progressed in Alzheimer's disease to participate. If Kathi is focused on cancer treatment, she might not be involved. How much longer can Butch participate? Maybe we only have five from that generation and we will need fifteen from our generation.

The doctor tactfully says, "Remember, no one is being forced to contribute to this research. It is your individual decision. It is not your family alone that shoulders this burden. There are other families out there already participating in research."

Silence falls across the room. The white tile floor is squared off with silver lines. I see my water bottle next to my chair and reach for it.

Seated by the window in the conference room, a cousin tries to understand our options. "The first scenario is that we line up, get blood drawn, and we never see you guys for the rest of our life. It helps you in research some, or maybe it doesn't, but I will never come back here again and I am done with it. That's one—"

An uncle interrupts in a sing-song tone, "That is one, but that is not the one you are going to do."

Laughter follows.

A deep voice cutting through the laughter is another uncle trying to keep us focused. "The second scenario is you give blood, you agree to do research and you come back every year, not here, but to NIH. You go through the lumbar puncture, the blood, the cognitive testing, just for the research. Then there is a third scenario, where you do all of that and you want to know, you get genetic testing and find out your status."

Another relative chimes in. "And there is a fourth, which is you do all the research, you don't want to know, but you then go for the genetic counseling because somebody else might want to know and their status affects you and you will still have to deal with it emotionally."

A person from the older generation who rarely speaks up says, "Then there is a fifth." His strong arm flinches as he talks. "The fifth is if your kids have it," he shakes his finger at the first cousin who talked about scenario number one, "then there is an opportunity for your kids to be healed by this disease, and if you don't go through it, someone else over here is going to go through it," he points across the room, "and you are going to owe them something at some point in your life, because they spent their time and their energy because of the main goal: they want to heal your kids and their kids and the wider world from the presence of Alzheimer's disease. So there is a major goal involved and it is healing the disease—it is killing the disease before it keeps going so we don't have to be here again. I will probably be long gone, but the positive end is ending the disease."

Gretchen Taylor, the NIH nurse who helped with Mom last year at the Memory Ride, speaks up for the first time. "Be careful you don't draw a wedge between your family. Respect each other's decisions, even if they are not the same as yours."

Dr. Watson adds, "I vividly recall the sounds of going to the nursing home to visit my great-great-grandmother." He points to his own chest. "I still have the heebie jeebies when I go into nursing homes. If you were a child when you first started seeing this illness, you will have a different perception of this than someone who is older." He motions to the youngest and older Noonan siblings, who have nearly a 20-year age difference. "This is well documented in other illnesses, that all of you have a different take on it, and that is how you cut each other some slack. Because what each of you see is a view based on the age of your eyes, the age of your brain, where you are in life at the time.

"Many of you by the time you were ten had changed a lot of diapers [on younger siblings]. It is very different and it robs you of different aspects of your life."

Dr. Watson pauses. "Now, the whole prospect of being able to get a genetic test to tell you whether you are going to go down that same path and be a burden, be aggressive, embarrass your family—these are the things that it conjures up. It doesn't have to be true, but that is the way you might have experienced it. You have to take that into consideration, to see if you really want to know. It is a complex process, to say the least."

After a short bathroom and snack break the conference resumes. I spent most of my break on my mini voice recorder summing up the conversations and my emotions. My legs are tight from sitting, my mind is full of information, and my heart is heavy.

"What prompted this [blood draw] today is that someone said, 'You better bring stuff to get my blood, cuz you might not get it again.'" Dr. Watson says.

He continues, "So, we came 'loaded for bear.' Giving blood today is not a necessity; it is more of an underscoring of one's intent to participate. What we have to figure out at some point is if we will get a number of people who are going to make this research study doable. This is not an easy fight. It is daunting, but the more power you get through numbers, the better off you are."

At this point, a cousin turns his wheelchair to face the two youngest cousins in the room, who have been agonizing over the lumbar puncture and blood draw. He is a metatropic dwarf who has been in a wheelchair all his life and is only three feet tall if you could stretch out his tight, curved body. He shakes his hands up and down three inches, his entire range of motion, to emphasize what he is going to say. "I've had a lot of experience getting my blood drawn, so if anybody wants me to take their blood—" he is interrupted by laughter. Loosey-goosey boney fingers wrap around the joystick that controls his wheelchair. His wide smile covers his entire face. His chuckles sound like gasping due to his fused vertebrae that compress his lung capacity.

"He draws blood with his teeth," a female cousin yells out.

The lecture is over and people are beginning to mingle. One uncle is making dinner reservations for interested family members. I wonder if I will be able to eat.

I take a seat at a round table in the back of the room near the video cameras, the impromptu nurse's station for drawing blood.

Gretchen Taylor, the nurse from NIH, secures a rubber strap around my upper arm and tells me to flex my hand into a fist. I'm dizzy and overwhelmed. Quickly, she inserts the needle and blood pours into the attached vial.

The nurse removes the vial filled with my blood and adds a new one into which my crimson fluid flows. She rechecks the small plastic tubes to be sure they are assigned to me.

The doctors have cautioned us that no one knows the full impact of genetic testing. It is too new. I overhear simultaneous conversations in which family members are exploring the worst case scenarios: we may be denied health insurance, or in the future be forced to find out our status before gaining insurance coverage, or even face employment discrimination. Freedom from discrimination based on genetic status is not yet part of our civil liberties. I have already said too much to acquaintances and people in my community without realizing it by openly telling people about Alzheimer's in my family and that it seems to be genetically linked.

All this information is playing bumper cars in my mind. In the last two weeks since we found out about the gene, I applied and was accepted for long-term-care insurance. I wasn't sure that, after finding out all this information about my potential genetic status today, I would still be eligible without lying on the intake evaluation. However, now I have to keep the insurance until I find out my genetic status. Or if I never find out, I should keep it at least until I'm 60 and therefore beyond our family's early-onset Alzheimer's disease strike zone. With my limited budget at this point, it is already expensive.

A few of my relatives are on their hands and knees peering at the human genome map, an intricate tapestry showing the genes in our body. It is too big to fit on a table. One of the doctors is pointing at the gene in our family that has mutated. The nurse taking my blood puts a piece of cotton and a Band-Aid on the point where the needle was extracted from my flesh.

I feel simultaneously obligated and desperate to participate in the genetic studies for me and my family. It is our only hope. The blood draw isn't a problem for me, but a spinal tap? A lumbar puncture that has the chance to leave me paralyzed?

Do I want to know my results? Can I handle the results? What if others find out their results?

CHAPTER 31

Gray Matter

UNRESPONSIVE, MOM IS RUSHED to the hospital within a week of the Boston family meeting. The scans and testing indicate she probably had a grand mal seizure. The CT scan reveals she has little gray matter left in her brain, as most of it has atrophied. Dr. Whyzesol, the Alzheimer's specialist, had warned at a recent appointment that seizures do occur in this stage of Alzheimer's disease.

The testing also determines her thyroid is low, and that she has a urinary tract infection and yeast infection. Dan talks with the staff and signs the appropriate paperwork. Evidence of her decline is indicated on this paperwork. The staff member indicates that Mom appears "well over her stated age," while, upon her admission into the secure unit eight months prior, the paperwork said "she definitely looks no more than her stated age." She is 58.

The nurse says, "She can go home now. Do you want an ambulance to take her back?" Having taken an ambulance to the hospital, Mom hasn't moved on her own since her arrival.

"No, it will be alright," Dan says. When the skeptical nurse leaves, Dan says to Mom, "They are releasing you. We gotta get out of here." He begins to squat to prepare to take her body in his arms.

Dan's jaw drops as Mom pops up in bed and puts her feet on the ground. Hearing a commotion behind him, he continues, "Okay, Mom, stand up. It is time to go."

Mom stands up as an out-of-breath attendant arrives with a wheelchair. Mom's head comes only to Dan's chest, and she waits expectantly. With swift and smooth care, he slides his arms under Mom's, picking her up and easing her into the wheelchair. The staff member holding the wheelchair and others watching from afar stare at Dan with mouths agape in amazement.

Dan takes the wheelchair, nodding to the helpful attendant, and says, "Thanks." Shrugging his broad, strong shoulders, he wheels Mom past the flabbergasted staff.

Mom is slumped forward, the heavy mass of her skull suspended by her neck. The rise and fall of her chest is her only movement. She is in a wheelchair in the hallway of the care facility.

"Hey, Mom, it's Kate, how are you doing?" I brush a wisp of hair away from her eyebrow as I crouch in front of her.

Rubbing her knee, I say, "Mom, Mom."

Her eyelids remain closed and her wet lips are sagging open.

A caregiver with long brown hair pulled into a ponytail says, "How's Mo?"

"She isn't responding. Has she been like this for long?" I ask.

The caregiver strides to the wheelchair in which Mom's body is wavering, threatening a fall forward as gravity pulls her heavy cranium toward the floor. "Hey Mo," she yells, and then proceeds to pinch Mom's upper arm fat.

Mom recoils, slurring her words. "Llleave me aalone."

The caregiver pokes Mom's side as she says to me, "You have to wake her." Anger flares inside of me.

Mom's pupils flicker under their lids. "Don't thouch me."

"Your daughter is here to see you," she demands.

"It's okay," I say, thrusting my hand out to stop the prodding caregiver. "I don't mind her sleeping."

"Mom, you have been through a lot, let your body rest." Taking out my apricot-rose lotion, I massage her limp, boney fingers and soft palms.

I knock on the door to Mom's room; there is no answer. I silently open the door and see Mom's dormant mound. Her hospital bed, ordered by hospice, is scheduled to arrive today. I tiptoe to the far side of the room and crawl in next to her, taking the opportunity to snuggle in her double bed one last time.

She doesn't move.

In a whisper I say, "Good morning, Mom."

Without opening her eyes she responds, "Good morning, Katie."

I smile, beaming. *How did she know it was me? How did she remember my name?* We both fall asleep in a morning catnap.

When we wake, I notice her face is swollen. White salt lines, the remaining traces of sorrow, are on her cheeks.

I tell her, "I love you so much."

With a cracking voice she says, "I know." Scrunching up her face and letting out two belly breaths, she begins to whimper.

"I wish I could take your pain away," I say. Lately, she has been less talkative and she cries more.

She says, "It was okay. I'm okay."

✳

CHAPTER 32

In Lieu of Hugs

MOM IS SITTING IN a wheelchair facing the window. Leaves on the trees outside have turned amber, cherry red, and pumpkin orange. I'm kneeling on the floor near her, the open bedroom window behind me.

The outhouse odor has subsided since Mom has been in diapers. Therefore, the urine on the bathroom floor was from Mom missing the toilet and not her angry wailing roommate, as I had assumed.

Finding out my 58-year-old mother is incontinent is a blow to my mental construct of her. With our roles reversed, I'm like a parent identifying with my child—I'm embarrassed and shocked by her decline. I want to scold her, yet I know it is not her fault; so instead, I want to cover it up. She is too young for this.

The hospice chaplain is visiting with a small black Bible. He sits in Mom's wooden rocking chair. His kindness permeates the room. It is his first visit to meet Mom. I'm here to be sure Mom is okay with a new person interacting with her. I wonder if he will try to push religious beliefs on Mom.

The chaplain asks, "How many children do you have?"

Mom answers, "Ten of us."

I jump in. "There are ten of Mom's siblings, and there are six of Maureen's children; four of us are located in Ashland."

He continues to try to get to know Mom and says, "I understand you have suffered many losses recently; I'm sorry your husband passed away. That must have been difficult for you."

Mom cocks her head to the side and with a wrinkled brow states, "I don't have a husband. I have never been married." Abruptly, Mom looks straight ahead, seemingly annoyed at the insinuation.

The chaplain has turned toward me. My mouth is gaping open. There is no way I will correct or clarify that answer. I learned from an article Dad gave me not to push the memories of death on someone with Alzheimer's disease. If she doesn't remember the pain, it seems like a blessing. However, I'm stunned.

He begins asking about Mom's religious background. I breathe a sigh of relief that he is catering to her individual spiritual needs, rather than his interpretation of what she needs to get into heaven.

I look at the brown, tan, and white Wal-Mart knit booties on Mom's feet, one of the many helpful suggestions of her sister Julie. *What is she going to say to this question?*

Mom answers, "Roman Catholic." Shocked, I stare back and forth between Mom and the chaplain. Mom is full of surprises.

I speak up again. "Well, she has most of the bases covered. She was Roman Catholic growing up. Mom and Dad moved to Iowa and got involved in the charismatic movement for awhile. Then, Dad went to seminary and became the pastor of a conservative Baptist church in a small town in New York state. After Dad left the parsonage, they attended a liberal Bible Mennonite church in Woodville, New York. And finally, I like to think of her as my little Buddha, as she forces me to be present in each moment."

Mom looks at me with dancing eyes and a huge, playful smile. I glance at the chaplain, not knowing what to expect. She is engaging me, but ignoring the chaplain. She is leaning forward. I push myself off my butt and onto my knees. It seems she wants something, but isn't asking for it. I keep watching her every move as she inches closer to me. Her lower body remains still; she seems to have lost the ability to move her arms, as she no longer gives hugs.

I'm aware the chaplain is here to visit with Mom, not to watch us interact. Mom doesn't seem to care or notice. She bends forward from her waist and I move to meet her, thinking she might fall out of her new hospice wheelchair if she leans any farther. I place my hands on the cold silver metal posts of her wheelchair and steal a nervous glance at the chaplain, who is peacefully watching. I shift, uneasy at the close proximity of Mom's face, but I stay engaged.

Mom's full grin is pulling out my own smile. Inches from me, she tilts her brow closer to me by pulling her chin in and pushing her white crown of hair in my direction. *What is she doing?* I reposition myself, unsure of what is taking place. It is as if she is drawing me in energetically with her fixed pupils. I try to resist, feeling both awkward with someone nearby and obligated to amuse her.

Then, she leans more and I reciprocate slowly. I feel the heat and then her baby-fine hair tickles my skin. Our foreheads softly touch, barely noticeable, and then with firmer pressure. Mom holds still; we are completely connected. As I breathe in, my shoulders drop. Our eyes close and a peaceful love comes over me. Flashes of heat flow from my head into the rest of my body. We hold the nurturing position for several minutes.

As slowly as we came together, we move apart. She smiles at me again. I smile in awe that she has found a way to connect physically with me. I'm sitting on my heels again with my right hand holding Mom's left. As a teardrop of joy trickles down my face, I turn to include the chaplain in our circle of quiet intimacy. Misty-eyed, he speaks slowly, respectful of what we share. He tells us in a low whisper, "That was beautiful."

✳

CHAPTER 33

Secret Costumes

Names omitted

STUFFING THE CURLY BLONDE wig, the raccoon costume, and the spectacles with attached rubbery nose and mustache into the overflowing black garbage sack, we clear off the dusty beige couch. Folding chairs have been set up in the far corner of the garage. The kids are with babysitters upstairs in the main house. Traffic noise filters into the secret cave-like meeting we are holding in Jay's basement.

After my siblings and our significant others are seated, the first person begins talking. "I'm going to do a quick recap so we are all on the same page. Speak up if there is anything you don't know, or add whatever I leave out.

"When Mom was transported to the emergency room two weeks ago for shaking spells and a possible seizure, a CAT scan revealed significant brain atrophy. The hospital staff was surprised Mom was functioning so well, as she had little gray matter remaining. Mom was given Rocephin, an antibiotic, for a urinary tract infection, and an IV with two liters of saline solution, as she was dehydrated—"

With arms folded across chest, a sibling interrupts, "Didn't the hospital ask if she wanted antibiotics? Was it to keep her alive longer or for physical pain?"

"Our family hadn't talked about it and was not prepared for her rapid decline. The hospital told me it was the normal protocol, so that is what I did." The original speaker shrugs, voice tight and defensive.

The sibling who interrupted sits back in the chair and nods knowingly.

As if upping the ante of a card game, a person adds, "Mom has lost fifty pounds in the last four months and hasn't been eating on her own."

Removing a chewed pen from mouth, a sibling queries, "At what point did the staff at Chapford begin feeding her? How long has it been?"

The original speaker responds, "They began giving her finger foods early this month. She needed reminders to eat in the past couple of months, although she wasn't consuming much."

Taking off a pair of brown dress shoes, another person adds, "I think nutritional drinks started last week."

The original speaker pulls a stack of papers from a bag. "We have been operating on immediate crisis mode. I think we need to ask a number of questions. Are we doing what we said we would do? Are we honoring her end-of-life wishes? Have we neglected to see the whole picture? Given Mom's drastic deterioration, I have been reviewing her living will and I think we need to make some clear, swift decisions." The voice is businesslike and this sibling begins to pass around photocopies of Mom's advance directive.

The documents reads, *I have made my feelings known to my agent(s) about artificial nutrition and hydration and I hereby give authority to said agent(s) to make any and all decisions about artificial nutrition and hydration.*

I signed and agreed to follow Mom's wishes at age 22, before she actually needed me to act as alternate power of attorney and health care proxy. "Alternate" was the standard precaution that I assumed we would never need. Alternate to Dad, whom I never imagined would die first. Biting my lip to hold back tears, I flip through the familiar documents.

When I moved to Kentucky, I was replaced as power of attorney and health care proxy by another sibling. Relieved of the duties, I was grateful not to be burdened by that intensity, but here I sit, nonetheless, poring over the intricate meaning of these documents.

"I wish it was written out, exactly what she wanted," the sibling who replaced me as Mom's power of attorney utters, while meticulously combing each paragraph.

The living will continues: ... *these instructions apply if I am in a persistent vegetative state for more than 30 days or if I am permanently unconscious or in an incurable or irreversible mental or physical condition with no reasonable expectation of recovery, or if I am in any other similar condition. Under any such circumstances, I direct my attending physician to withhold or withdraw treatment that only serves to prolong the process of my dying and that I be allowed to die and not be kept alive by medical procedures, medications, artificial means (including, but not limited to, artificial feeding, hydration, and respiration)* ....

A person sitting on the beige couch suggests, "If she is swallowing the food, then it could be argued that she wants to eat and is simply unable to lift the spoon."

One person chews on a hangnail. A few people are motionless. The person in one of the folding chairs is tapping a heel against the metal crossbar, making an annoying sound that accelerates in tempo as emotions start to heat up over our family's discussion.

Heads rapidly swivel to the beanbag chair as the next person begins talking. "I disagree; I have fed her and don't think she really wants to eat. We are caught up in having her eat because it is ingrained in us, feeling like we are nurturing and caring for her with food. She has been spitting food out. If she can't verbally communicate with us, at least we can pay attention to the nonverbal cues and previous wishes."

From the couch, a soft voice speaks. "Lifting her spoon and giving her nutritionally enriched drinks seems to be crossing the line. They serve only to prolong the inevitable."

Unbuttoning a sage green work shirt, a person stands up to take it off, revealing a white t-shirt with wet-stained armpits. This person hooks the collar of the dress shirt over the pantry door. Turning back to the group, "You know she will die fairly quickly if she is no longer taking in food?"

Despite the obvious truth of this statement, it hangs in the air. What is left unsaid is that we are influencing the timing of her death.

Tears form and roll down the next speaker's face. "That is the hardest part."

Scooting forward on the metal folding chair, another person reaches out and touches the knee of the crying sibling while asking, "What is underneath that? Do you need more time with Mom? Are you afraid to let her die?"

"Ummm ... I didn't know it would happen so soon. I mean, in some ways it has been the longest couple of years of my life and I thought it would last a while longer, but suddenly it's almost over," the speaker mumbles through a tissue.

Quiet, lonely angst pauses the discussion for a moment.

A hushed but determined voice continues the conversation. "Let me acknowledge that I hate that we have to discuss this. I miss who Mom used to be." Pausing for a moment, this person makes eye contact with the teary sibling before resuming. "The course has been slippery. It is now or never to speak up. Already, we allowed the hospital to administer antibiotics and an IV without realizing she was at this stage. And Chapford, using its normal protocol, has been forcing nutritional drinks. It is time to stop. Her life will not improve anymore."

Squinting and scratching behind an ear, a person says, "I may be as much to blame as Chapford. I bought her children's re-hydration purple liquid and sippy cups designed for toddlers to make it easier for her to drink without spilling. Stepping back to see the whole picture, my premise of trying to keep her hydrated so she doesn't go to the hospital is incorrect."

"Do you think she is really done here?" a musing voice wonders aloud. This person has been fairly quiet the whole meeting.

Annoyed, a person seated on the couch replies with a chastising voice, "If you are talking about her soul's quest in this life, I don't believe that is for us to determine. We need only determine when and how to follow her living will." Then, as if giving in to the question, this person says with a softened tone, "But I think she is complete. She has been holding on to help solve the mystery of Alzheimer's and once the scientists detected the Alzheimer's gene in our family, she was ready to let go. There is nothing more she can do to help. It doesn't seem inconsequential that her decline immediately followed the discovery of the gene associated with our family's Alzheimer's plague."

Faces around me are pale—I'm guessing matching my own. I hear my family's voices weaving back and forth trying to come to an agreement of how to handle Mom's request, yet none of us want to play God. A cold sweat is building on my palms and back. Autumn drafts push into the basement from under the garage door, stirring up dust off the Ping-Pong table.

"I don't know if I can do it," one person says, two hours into our discussion.

"Even if she has entrusted you with her best interest?" With disbelief, a different voice pipes into this segment of the conversation.

"Well, what is in her best interest? Mom always protected me whenever she thought I was hurt. Am I doing the same for her by letting her die sooner—or am I doing the same for her if I make sure she digests food if she is hungry? Am I making decisions based on what I would want in her situation, rather than what she actually wants? Is there any chance that in her new state of being with Alzheimer's, her death wishes have changed?" the person replies, snuggling deeper into a blanket wrapped around shoulders.

Abruptly, a person slouching in a folding chair lengthens to a full upright position. "You're joking, right?" With full-bodied emotion, the loud, sharp interjection continues. "I want to make it crystal clear to all of you right now, my death wishes and living will are not going to change if I get Alzheimer's. If anything, they will become stronger."

Another sibling jumps into the conversation. "Yeah, now I know who NOT to have as my power of attorney." The words are punctuated by a bitter laugh tinged with utter sadness.

The laughter rings in the room. My mind races thinking about my own fate and the fate of my siblings. We are absorbed in thought. Closing my eyes for a brief second, I say a silent prayer for our collective future.

With a diffused tone, the person in the middle of the couch says, "If I was in her spot, I wouldn't want to be there and I would hope that someone would examine what I asked for and honor it."

The apparent defendant in this conversation crosses arms in

front of chest. Serene but powerful, the voice responds, "If you are specific in your living will, I will honor whatever you want. At this point, I'm not certain that Mom wants to die. The problem I'm having with Mom's will is that she wasn't explicit given all the new scenarios."

"No one can determine what scenarios will be present at their time of death. That is why the following clause is incorporated," says a sibling with a lawyer-like voice, pausing to flip through the living will ditto sheets. "*I hereby give authority to said agent(s) to make any and all decisions about artificial nutrition and hydration.*" Putting down the sheets, the sibling continues. "If we knew all the scenarios, no one would need a health care proxy. I believe honoring Mom's living will means letting her die. We have violated her advance directive already. However, I'm willing to wait to institute her living will until all of you are ready to let her go. It is a one-way process and once we stop feeding her, we can't go back and forth. The longer we wait the harder it will be to do this and the more opposition we will see from Chapford."

"That is a good point; we need to be careful here," one of the older siblings shares. "I don't want us to be like the Noonan family at their mother's funeral." This person is talking about our mother's siblings and the death of our grandmother, Julia Tatro Noonan, in 1978. "Half of the family wanted her to be buried with rosary beads because she used to be Catholic, but the other siblings did not want rosary beads because they were now Baptist and thought it would influence her spirit's path after death. Their anger lingered long after her death and impacted their relationships."

In unison several of us exclaim, "I have never heard that before."

Another sibling chimes in. "That's ironic—I heard recently the Noonan siblings have volunteered Grandma's grave to be dug up if her DNA would be of assistance to help researchers in the fight to track the gene and end Alzheimer's in our family."

Hearing it vocalized, I shudder, thinking about the dirt piles that were waiting to cover my father's casket. And I wonder about Grandma, her burial plot, skeleton bones, baggy clothes that no longer fit, and scientists taking samples. I look at my family members in the room, waiting impatiently for someone to talk, to change my morbid thought pattern.

"I agree that our relationships with each other are more important than Mom's wishes at this juncture. She is going to die either way." This sibling makes visual contact with everyone in the room before continuing. "But don't get me wrong—I feel strongly that the right thing is to quit feeding her altogether."

"I'm not ready to stop all food. I need to think about it," a sibling with blazing cobalt eyes launches into the debate. "The only thing I know for certain is that she doesn't want an IV or tube feeding. Everything else is a bit ambiguous. It's confusing. Where is the cutoff point?" The person begins to count off options on fingers. "One, don't continue to bring food to Mom if she isn't eating. Two, bring her food. Put it in front of her, but don't bring it to her mouth. Let her eat if she is able to on her own."

Ticking another finger, the sibling continues. "Three, lift food to her mouth. If she refuses it, then don't continue offering it. Four, lift the food to her mouth, force it between her lips. If she spits it out, quit feeding her. Five, if she isn't eating much, then put liquid nutrients in her cup." Switching to the fingers of the other hand, the speaker says, "Six, if she can't hold her own cup, then lift it for her." Then, shrugging shoulders and holding open both hands, the exasperated and weary sibling inquires, "Finally, at what point does the caregiver stop the protein drinks and start a feeding tube and an IV?"

A dog barks from the neighbor's yard, reminding me there is life outside of this decision. I take a deep breath. We are all here to honor Mom's wishes. Looking at my siblings, it is as if we are all transparent. Sorrow, loss, and emptiness present themselves uniquely in each of us: tight lips, glossy eyes, a stiff body, sunken cheeks, the furrowed brow or a hoarse voice. Exhaustion is mutual—mentally, due to mulling this over in our minds, and physically, from spending so much time in these meetings that eat away our free time, personal family time, and sleep.

From the couch a person responds to the scenarios. "Obviously, we process things differently, I get that. Some of us glance at the issue and can make quick decisions—not necessarily the best decision. But bam, it is done. While others of us intently contemplate the issue, pick it apart, put it back together, discuss all the options, analyze different scenarios, prepare backup plans for all the scenarios, and sit with how each decision will feel. I don't have the patience or energy to process like you and you'd feel rash and irresponsible if you processed like me."

With a raised eyebrow, a skeptical voice inquires, "How did you reach your decision?"

"There has been a decrease in her quality of life. On the days she is unresponsive, it's sort of like a coma and that haunts me," this sibling says sullenly. "Especially because Mom used to talk about when her mom was in a nursing home with IVs and a feeding tube, curled up in the fetal position. Grandma wouldn't respond when Mom came into the room. Sometimes she would move her foot to the music of a piano that was playing in another room. Mom didn't say it in these words, but the implication was that she didn't want to be kept alive for the few times that she was able to recognize a tune and tap her foot; it wasn't worth it to her. And clearly, the one thing that kept the process going on inevitably for Grandma was that she was force fed."

Passionately, the speaker continues, using hands to emphasize the words. "Put together Mom's lack of interaction, what we learned from the brain scan, her inability to eat, and her precipitous decline—in everything she conveyed, she didn't want to be in the state she is in right now."

Captivated by the speaker's passion, everyone waits for the next words. The speaker touches index finger to edge of mouth, gathering thoughts. After a moment, the index finger moves purposefully forward as words resume. "It isn't one event for me, but all those things. I don't see a meaningful reason for her to stay around; there is no redeeming piece. She clearly said to me, 'don't feed me; I don't want to be fed.' Whether or not she is getting nutrients by being hand fed, nutritional drinks, or a feeding tube doesn't matter; it's all nit-picking. The essence is the same. Everything is lined up, everything that needs to fall has fallen for me to make this decision. None of the dominoes remain standing at this point."

Hushed silence follows, but there is a tingling in my ears, similar to the sound of carbonation in soda pop. I wonder if I'm hearing the electrified movement of my cerebral spinal fluid stirring in my vertebrae, the very liquid that holds my DNA.

The same speaker sympathetically asks, "How much time do you need to make a decision? A day or a couple of weeks?"

Rubbing a tummy, a sibling responds, "I think two days. I need to be sure I can live with myself if we do this."

A voice questions, "You make it sound like it isn't her wishes. Do you think we are going against her will?"

Hesitating, this sibling discloses, "I'm not sure. She still has some good moments in the context of her life. I understand we are in a hurry to take action, but I need forty-eight hours."

"I'm more on the fence also. It feels so drastic."

"Take as much time as you need. This is a big decision. It would be a tragedy if you can't live with the decision once it is made."

A number of heads nod in agreement.

Nothing more is said. The emotional voltage and sense of confusion is palpable in the room. We exchange hugs in silence.

As we are going up the basement stairs into Jay's home, I can hear Jay's children greeting each person as he or she emerges into the large, airy living room. Gleeful, the children stomp and yelp as they grab onto legs and are lifted up into familiar arms for hugs. Everything shifts, and the heaviness of the basement discussion settles.

However, their joy makes me lighter, yet sadder. *Will these children be involved in end-of-life decisions for us?* Researchers tell us that in five years they will have made significant progress. My aunt tells me that the researchers have been saying "five years" for ten years already. *Is it too much to hope that all of us will escape having the Alzheimer's gene?*

CHAPTER 34

Killing Your Mother

Names omitted

TWO DAYS LATER, OUR meeting continues. Again, we are in the basement garage. This time, rain is pattering at the windows. Each one of us is haggard from more stress and less sleep. Gray hair is multiplying on our youthful heads and dark encircles our eyes.

Silently, I whisper one of my prayers. *Please, give Mom peace, love, joy, self-acceptance, and the rest of us wisdom, deep wisdom.*

One sibling begins. "After our last meeting, I went to Chapford to see for myself Mom's demeanor at mealtime. She wasn't interested in dinner. But I watched a staff member feed another resident. The old woman was choking on the food because the caregiver wasn't paying attention and kept cramming food into her mouth! It made me realize that Chapford's intent is to keep the occupants alive. I doubt they will be able to follow Mom's wishes to let go."

Nodding from the couch a person says, "I mentioned the living will to some of the staff at Chapford. They implied we are—" the voice trembles as it continues, "killing her."

Another person interjects, "It's a societal thing to try and keep people alive."

"The reality is that most people who go into a care facility die there," a sibling explains. "The subtext is they are losing money if someone dies. And they make money—thousands of dollars a month times the number of months they are able to get nutrition into her and keep her lingering on."

"How do we come to terms with the staff at Chapford treating us like we are killing our own mother? It is strange that they would think our love for her and commitment to her living will is homicide."

"Obviously, this is an unusual case. Mom's living will does not explicitly state not to bring a spoon to her mouth, although some of us heard her say that. We will have to sit down with them and discuss what we believe Mom wants."

"Chapford doesn't care about how we feel Mom would want to be treated. It is a business and they need concrete evidence to treat her any different than their normal protocol. If we are wishy-washy, Chapford will not honor it. We have to be definite and united. Ideally, we want Mom to stay there. It would be the easiest option, but we can't let her live there if they continue to feed her."

"Do we all agree this is what she would want and it is time to enforce her living will? Have we reached that decision?"

No one is moving; it is as if we are all holding our breath, waiting like a jury to deliver our individual decisions and thereby reach the final result of our deliberations.

"I'm not as positive as you. I feel Mom would agree, but I never had those conversations with her. I don't know if I will ever think either choice is the right decision. I hope that I'm following her wishes. On some level, I have to trust you, what you remember Mom saying, and your surety that the timing to implement her living will is now."

With a scrunched forehead and chin resting on hand, a sibling replies, "I don't quite follow what you are saying."

Like a teeter-totter, the speaker's head rocks from side to side, weighing the decision. "I will go along with this decision, but it is still hard for me. I do trust all of you, so the essence of my decision is based on that trust."

Rain drones on, *tititititititititititititititititit*, combining drops from the gutter, *dop dop dop dop dop dop*, dulling any other sound.

A sibling asks, "How will Mom's siblings perceive this? Do we need to include them?"

"It doesn't matter what they think. They are not in charge of her living will; we are. However, I think they would be completely supportive."

"Why don't you call some of them to find out?"

Aunt Julie's firm voice responds to our concerns through the telephone receiver. "I can assure you. Your mother and her siblings would not want to be kept alive in her condition. It is the product of being the second generation with Alzheimer's disease. We watched our mother deteriorate so slowly it was painful. It is similar to how you will feel after coming through your mother's illness. I believe you will not want to be kept alive either. Our society values life to the extent that we are denied death even when our time has come." There is a slight pause as Julie continues in a softened tone. "It is difficult and I'm so sorry you're facing this situation. Her time has come; let her go."

Reassured, we take a ten-minute break. I take full, deep breaths after hearing Julie's response. I step outside into the dark night and the rain hits my face, cooling it with each drop.

Returning to the basement, I pick a new seat.

Tentative, a sibling glances around the room. "One family member who lives in Massachusetts agrees that 'Mo would not want to be fed,' but wants us to keep giving her artificial nutrition until the rest of the extended family can come out to visit if they so desire."

"If we tell Chapford not to feed her, we can't go back on our word and ask them to keep feeding her for the time being. And the longer we wait to tell Chapford not to feed her, the harder it will be to implement and convince them to stop feeding her," snaps a sibling with a furrowed brow.

The sibling relaying the information says, "The family member wants us to sneak in protein drinks without Chapford knowing."

The furrowed brow moves into deep creases, with squinty, focused eyes. "What the fuck? That's ridiculous. After all of these conversations, I will not sneak drinks." Incensed, the person continues, "Let that person do it themselves. The relatives know she is rapidly declining. If they want to see her, they should get out here—she is dying."

Raising open palms, attempting to stop or calm the angry sibling who just spoke, the messenger replies, "Hey, don't get pissed at me. I didn't say it was a good idea; I'm simply passing on the information. That person is not going to fly out and do it—too busy with work—but the person thinks it is a good idea that one of us does it."

The rain continues in a steady downpour.

Three days later, I search through Mom's belongings in the dusty attic of the large, metal barn. I'm gathering items for a closing ceremony. It will be a collective remembrance, an appreciation of Mom's life, and a blessing of her passage into the dimensions beyond. Finding objects to decorate her room at Chapford, I'm attempting to represent all aspects of her life, including pictures, tools, her squad jacket, favorite jewelry, fancy dress shoes, work gloves, the Bible with plastic tabs and a navy zippered cover, her handwriting, and lilac perfume.

Inside a rectangular tomato box, I find a stack of cards that Mom has kept over the years. Dad was always the sentimental one, and Mom was the more practical one who threw away excess clutter. I'm surprised she chose to keep some notes, and doubly surprised they survived her numerous trips to the dump. Inside one particular card that has a basket of flowers on the front cover, I see my own writing. *She kept a note from me!*

I have thought a lot about what you asked of me a couple of weeks ago. You requested that I ensure your desires concerning medical treatment be implemented. I will do that for you. I'm glad you feel comfortable with me to ask me to do this.

Holding the card to my chest, I recline onto the wood plank flooring. My body relaxes for the first time in weeks. Taking a breath, I whisper, "Thank you," as a tear trickles into my ear.

*

CHAPTER 35

Scorn of Chapford

Names omitted

STANDING IN THE PARKING lot outside the locked care facility, my siblings and I sign copies of the letter that we have revised numerous times in the past week. I'm wearing black pants and a black shirt with a royal blue silk scarf slung around my neck. It is the color of the throat chakra and associated with speaking one's truth. I'm dressed up, yet all my bare nerves are showing.

Walking past the fake gas fireplace into the formal meeting area, we enter the same room we visited nine months prior where we asked questions about the facility and its philosophy on Alzheimer's disease. They had sold us then; it was by far the best situation for Mom. At the time, they said that they would honor her living will.

The room's wallpaper is a purpled maroon, from the floor boards to the chair rail. The remainder of the wall is off-white. We gather again around the oval wooden table, this time with the addition of Chantel, a nurse from hospice.

As we close the French doors behind us, the meeting with the director of the facility and the building supervisor commences. One sibling begins. "First, we want to thank you for the kindness your staff has shown to our mother. And secondly, we want to discuss with you Maureen's current condition and her living will."

Another sibling speaks. "In September, Mom took fewer bites and the staff fed her more bites. It happened so gradually we barely noticed. After Mom's stroke and the brain scans, which showed very little gray matter, her interest in eating dwindled further. Then, we realized she was being fed nutritional drinks to supplement her food intake. Her drastic decline caught us off-guard, but now we recognize where Mom is headed. In the next stage she will have difficulty swallowing, then comes the IVs and nutrition throat tubes that Mom's mother tolerated. It is the very scenario Mom hoped to avoid. She does not want to be artificially fed—"

The director of the facility interrupts. "It isn't artificial feeding because the staff members are only lifting a spoon. We are simply helping her out when she needs to be helped."

Another sibling reads from the living will. "*Withhold or withdraw treatment that only serves to prolong the process of my dying.*"

The director states, "I will continue to feed Mo as long as she is under my care; she is still eating and seems hungry."

An exasperated sibling retorts, "Have you tried feeding her yourself? She has little interest in food and often spits food out if someone puts it into her mouth."

Chantel from hospice sits forward. "Do you mind if I add something here?"

"No, please go ahead," the sibling replies, yielding the floor and taking a frustrated breath.

"Swallowing is an automatic response, like breathing. When food is put in her mouth, she can swallow, choke, or spit it out. If she does consume morsels, I don't believe it means that she is craving food, but rather, acting from an unconscious, instinctive reaction."

The director squints at Chantel. "Have you ever dealt with a similar situation, where a family refuses to feed a vulnerable and defenseless incapacitated family member?"

One of us interrupts. "We don't think of her as defenseless; she declared the living will when she had a clear mind."

Chantel continues to dissipate the energy and keep the conversation focused. "We encounter all kinds of situations. This is different from what I have been involved with as the instructions and wishes of Mo are proactive and preventative, given the genetic aspect of her disease, and having watched her mother artificially fed. I'm impressed by the strength and cohesiveness of this family. At hospice we believe that dying is part of life, a completing of the cycle, and that it need not be feared but can be walked into with power, dignity, and respect. Mo is doing exactly that and we are supportive of the Preskenis family ensuring quality of life rather than a prolonged life."

The director drums the table with her extra-long painted fingernails and says, "My staff is doing a fine job ensuring she is healthy." Visibly shaking, she steals a disconcerted glance at the building supervisor, who is still as a statue with her hands folded.

The family member sitting closest to the director states, "Yes, we agree the staff wants Mo to be healthy and they are kind to her. We appreciate that. However, at this stage, Mo doesn't want to be fed or, for that matter, consuming nutrition that she can't feed herself. She doesn't want to prolong her life."

Another sibling explains with a firm voice, "We—Mo's children—hospice, and Dr. Whyzesol believe she is in her final stage of life and is preparing for her death. This isn't about killing her, but allowing death in her natural time frame."

Another sibling says, "We request that you tell your staff to stop feeding Mo and to not give her any more nutrient-enriched drinks. Will you honor this request?"

"What you are asking me to do is negligence! I can't kill Mo." The director stops as her face contorts, and then in a high-pitched voice she continues, as if flipping personalities, "I won't allow it to happen. Oh—Mo, Mo, *mmmh* Mo." She begins to bat her watery eyelids.

My siblings and I look at each other in confusion over the director's bizarre behavior. Silence settles over the room. Out of the bay window, I notice vibrant green ivy is crawling up the grayish brick wall near the walkway.

Why is she crying? Is she trying to fake concern for Mom? She doesn't have much personal interaction with Mom. Why the strong reaction? Is this the reality of business? Losing a resident affects income and therefore her emotions?

As we wait for the director to compose herself, I realize that Chapford needs to keep people alive for job security. The more nutrition they can cram down her, the longer that money will be guaranteed. If Mom is allowed to die at this stage, what kind of precedent would that set?

On the edge of my chair, I feel energy gushing through my nerves. Wrapped up in the meeting, I feel the intense opposition and the implication that we are killing Mom. My mouth quivers from frown to smile, frown, smile—uncontrollable flickering. I almost start to laugh but nothing is funny; in fact, it is so serious, I feel a bit like a maniac, out of control. I draw in a sip of cool water from my Nalgene to keep the edges of my mouth still. Then I fill my lungs with air, forcing my spine against the upholstered chair. Clenching the arms of the chair, I hold my body tight to the seat cushion and grit my teeth.

"Mumggh." Clearing her throat, the director talks in her normal voice. "I will report to the State that she is leaving our facility. It is my duty to report such occurrences. They will take it from there."

Her words reach across the table, grabbing our throats. Fear pulses in unison between us. *Will the district attorney come knocking on our door?*

The building supervisor suspiciously inquires, "Where will you be moving her?"

"We have been communicating with one foster home and they have done the initial evaluation of Mom. We hope to make the transition within two weeks."

"Did that home agree to follow this … this … this request to not feed Mo?" the director asks with skepticism.

I turn away from the director and look at the sibling seated next to me. I roll my eyes. This sibling rubs my back. I'm exhausted. After this whole discussion, the director still doesn't understand quality of life versus quantity of days. I don't want to disclose any details about Mom's future home. The sibling firmly cups my shoulder with a palm.

The meeting is over. Some of my siblings go out to the parking lot with Chantel. A couple of us want to see Mom before we leave. The director and the building supervisor go into an office.

Mom sat oblivious to the meeting less than forty feet away in the living room behind the locked maroon door. After pressing the code on the keypad, a few of the siblings enter the room where she sits. She is in a wheelchair at a round table with dinner in front of her. We give her a hug and say hello, and she responds with garbled words. "Glad to seeee …" before her voice trails off. She stares into space and then at her slippers, never gazing at the steaming hot mashed potatoes.

Muffled rustling comes from the area behind me. For the first time, I notice that the wall is actually a window with a curtain on the other side. A hand brushes the large curtain open, making it seem like the wall is giving way, exposing this window I hadn't realized existed. Bright light from the internal office that the window reveals streaks into the dining area.

Stunned, I step back. Two stern women, their faces long and stressed, peer out of the glass. This side of the window is my mom and siblings in the locked facility; that side of the window is the director and supervisor in an office. An uncanny sensation swoops across my body.

To add to our anxiousness, Mom takes a bite.

The building supervisor pulls a chair close to the window and the facility director perches on the desk with one leg dangling while she crosses her arms over her chest. Obvious surveillance. There are cameras all around the unit monitoring the residents, staff, and visitors. This is an intentional power portrayal. Like a little mouse under a hawk, I avert my gaze and scurry away from the piercing, electrifying stares, huddling near Mom.

It is the most awkward game of apparent control I have ever witnessed. Mom glances away, not paying attention to her food. Minutes later, the glassed observers gain the lead as she notices the meal and takes a feeble bite, but we intercept the touchdown as the morsel drops on her slipper. She doesn't care, but simply glances away. Then Mom turns to us. Her Caribbean-blue eyes light up as if seeing us for the first time. In slurred words she says, "I love yoou."

CHAPTER 36

Opening My Home

Names omitted

EXCITEDLY, I SPURT OUT, "I have decided that I want to take Mom into my home."

I say this at the beginning of the family meeting that I have specifically requested since Chapford is unwilling to honor Mom's living will. A gigantic smile is on my face, as I'm speaking the truth of my internal knowing and alignment. Energy is racing through my body, simmering in my hands and feet. We are in Karen and Guy's home and I'm kneeling on the floor in front of the piano opposite their lime-green velour couch. The couch is part of the living room set that originally belonged to Guy's grandparents.

Caw caw, a crow flutters into the giant redwood outside of their home. Everyone is silent. One person looks down, another out the window, a couple of others stare at me with mouths agape.

Adjusting my posture, I sit erect. "You all think that I'm crazy. I would think you were crazy if you told me the same thing. I might be, but I have to try. It is important to honor Mom's living will and not only do I think I can have her in my home, I want her in my home."

"Have you talked to Jim about it?" the first voice asks.

"Yes, we realize it will be difficult, but he is supportive. This is a one-time opportunity and it isn't like she will be crazy with Alzheimer's wanderings or threatening anger."

"Why do you want to do this?" another voice questions. Divots riddle the speaker's forehead.

"I want to watch her go through the dying process. I missed Dad's, and the biggest thing I regret about his death is that I couldn't be part of it and witness it for him or help him through it." My reason remains solid.

"Why do you want her in your space?" This person is utterly confused and is sincerely trying to comprehend my thought process.

Closing my eyes for a moment to attempt a direct translation from my soul, I say, "I want to have her in my home. To do yoga, meditate, and sleep near her. I want to be close to Mom, feel her warm body and touch her."

"It seems to me you can do that with her in a foster home," a voice from the matching lime-green rocking chair observes. "Are there any other reasons why you want her in your space?"

"Well, I want to be able to cry about her dying without having to hush my grieving in the semi-public setting of a foster home, and I can crawl in bed with her anytime of the day or night. In another home, I'm not sure they would allow that."

A voice responds, "I don't think I would be at ease coming and going if Mom was in your home, even if you told me it was fine. I also don't think I would be as emotional with her in your space. I would rather have a neutral location."

"Really?" I ask in disbelief, shocked that what makes me comfortable would create the opposite effect for someone else, "I want you all to be as involved or uninvolved as you desire. And about processing your emotions, I would be happy to leave anytime you want."

"That is it," a sibling says in a direct but hushed tone, "I don't feel comfortable essentially kicking you out of your home."

Another person adds, "Since you and I are neighbors, having her in your home is way too close for me. With my luck and past history, even if she appears bedbound or on her deathbed, she will get up and walk on her own down to my house." The voice laughs and says, "Lazarus? Is that you?"

I smile, knowing that person might be right, but before I can respond, another voice chimes in. "What about you getting space you need away from Mom?"

Immediately I reply, "I don't think I need much space, as I'm planning on being with her most of the time, anyway. I have already told my work that I'm taking time off. I think we will be able to get twenty-four-hour care with a care-giving service, and it falls under her long-term-care insurance policy. I can always leave when a caregiver is working."

"Who will be responsible for her medications?"

As if I'm being interrogated by police, I cautiously reply, "The caregivers will be responsible for administering everything and hospice will be involved."

"From what I understand, hospice will not be around all the time. Are you willing to oversee the caregivers? They will be continually rotating through—there needs to be some sort of consistency," the person in the wood rocking chair says, as the branches of the Ficus tree behind the chair wiggle with each rock.

Another probes, "So if you are ultimately responsible, how would you feel if we ask you what is going on and question the medications or changes? How would you feel if one of us gets frustrated at you for not keeping up on one aspect of her care?"

Pinching my fingernails together, I pull at the tiny loops of carpet underneath me. I swallow hard. "That would be difficult for me. I'm a perfectionist and hate to have anyone angry with me, especially you guys. I know you would be asking about Mom, but I might take it as personal that you are criticizing me."

Another voice says, "Her medications will get more complicated as there needs to be constant monitoring of her increasing pain. We were coordinating so much of her physical care when she lived in the trailer and while at the original foster home, and then we placed her in Chapford and they took it on. I don't want to have to take any of that responsibility back."

I listen without saying a word. The room is stacked against me. I wonder if I should have taken a seat in a chair to have more apparent power, rather than sitting on the floor near the hallway.

"How would you feel if none of us are willing to assist you with her physical daily care?" This person's feet are crossed and hands are folded.

My jaw tenses. I'm tired of the questions. I want them to be supportive. "I don't know. I think I would be fine."

Another person interjects, "I wouldn't want you to be ultimately responsible for her care. I know you extremely well and feel when you are stressed. That would make me stressed, too, and I would feel obligated to step in to help even if I don't want to."

"Katie, what if she gets well again and begins to eat food on her own?" This person is asking the obvious question that all of us have been afraid to admit to each other, fearing it might actually happen. They are leaning forward, looking intently at me.

Blowing a big breath out of my lungs, with my lower lip curled over the top one, the air shoots to the top of my brows. "I do realize there are a couple of big unknowns and that is the biggest. Her current rate of activity fluctuates. One week she is up and well, and the next she is unresponsive and bedbound. What if she isn't dying?"

"Or what if it doesn't work to have her there?"

"I can't take care of her long term. I think if need be, I could have her in my space for two, maybe three months. Then, it would mean finding a different home for her."

Slumping in the corner of the couch, another person says, "I do not have the patience to move her again. I need this next move to be her last. It takes too much energy finding the home and planning the move and preparing the staff. If she died in your house, how would you feel continuing to live there?"

"I would be fine; I doubt she would haunt it, if that is what you mean. I want to be with her when she dies and will be grateful for the time I get to spend with her."

The room falls silent. We all look at each other.

Finally, a sibling's partner speaks. "We have covered the major details. Let's take a vote to see if it is a close decision and if we need to continue further deliberations. By a show of hands, who thinks it's a good idea for Mom to live and die at Kate's home?"

I raise my hand, but it is the only one in the air. I search each person's face to see if his or her decision is final. Each face is solemn. The vote is cast. I lower my lonely hand to rest on my abdomen. Then, I bring my other hand to my face and bite on the end of my thumbnail, trying to stabilize the tornado inside of me.

GNNNNNN, the buzzer sounds on a dryer in the adjacent laundry room, causing my body to jolt.

Defeated, I say, "I'm obviously outnumbered. I agree the health of our relationship to each other is the most important aspect of this entire situation. I will let it go."

"We love you, Katie. We want to respect your desire to do this, but we are exhausted. We need to do what is best for all of us." The voice is reassuring, but my insides are in volatile tangles.

"I'm frustrated, but understand," I say, acknowledging feeling cheated out of this potentially amazing experience, as well as comprehending the impact it would have on them.

Each one gives me a hug and I bite the inside of my lower lip. I spread open my eyelids and dab the corners with my knuckles so fluid won't accumulate on the rims and expose even more vulnerability. I don't want the dam to break here, not under these circumstances. I need space.

Upon leaving the family meeting, the rising floodwater and the nettling of my quivering chin break the dam. Tears gush forth. Given the amount of liquid that flows out of them, my eyes are virtually swollen shut by the time I reach my friend Jessica's yellow house. My vision is blurry and my chest is cramped. I collapse on her purple velvet bed, sobbing.

CHAPTER 37

Triumphant Stupor

AS MY SIBLINGS, UNCLE Eryc, and I move Mom's belongings into Beth's foster home, I toss my duffle bag stuffed with essentials in the huge walk-in closet off the bathroom, a place bedbound Mom will never see. Mom gets the expansive master bedroom, a private room in the back of the house.

Inside the duffle bag are a pillow, a sleeping bag, yoga gear, clothes, my journal, and books. I'm acutely aware that Mom, the forgetful, curious, exploring person with Alzheimer's disease, will not touch my things. She is beyond the stage of my needing to hide everything precious from her sight and reach. Now it is I who am prying as I stretch, maybe invasively, into her experience to glean insight about death and the other side. I'm planning to spend most nights with Mom until she passes, leaving whenever my siblings want space and when Jim and I need time together.

✳

Red and yellow leaves with green splotches float down from the nearby American Basswood tree. Old, crisp brown leaves rest on the deck. Cool autumn air floats in through the bedroom bay window. Mom has been in this foster home for a week.

Mom interrupts my dreamy state as she stutters, "I go. I am gonna go there. I go. I'm glad." Mom is teary and her voice quivers. "That's good. I want to get away from there. I don't want that."

I ask, "Are you sad?" trying to interpret her tears mixed with smiles.

Mom hastily says, "No" and then follows that with a quieter "Yeah."

"I get sad a lot, too," I reply. Then I take her hand in mine. It is hot and swollen, along with her right foot. *Why are only her right extremities swollen and not the left side?*

Out of nowhere Mom says, "I'll write it down."

Stunned by her words, and not sure what she is referring to, I promptly ask, "Do you want paper and a pen?"

Mom replies, "Yeah."

Fumbling through my purple bag, I rip sheets out of my journal and hand her my pen and paper. She doesn't seem coordinated enough to hold them, so I set them on the bedside table. I lower her left bed rail.

As I proceed to adjust the table to a height she will be able to write on, she continues in abstract sentences. "I don't care. I don't know exactly where he is going. This one here."

The bedside table wobbles as I maneuver it down and the white Bic pen rolls, gaining momentum. The speed of the pen carries it over the rubber edge of the table and toward Mom's bed.

Like lightning, her left hand snatches the pen out of the air. She holds it, tight fisted.

My eyes flare open and jawbone drops, leaving a wide chasm. Her hand appears like an athlete's in a triumphant exclamation of victory. Her face is expressionless as if nothing out of the ordinary has happened.

"You are fast," I exclaim in astonishment. "How did you grab it so quick?"

Mom replies casually, "I just said wha—I didn't think it was thinking." Mom sets the pen down on the ragged edge of blank journal paper that is on the bedside table and then returns her arm to her side. This is the table where her food is placed. *Mom has the physical mobility to eat food if she desired.*

Ghghghgnnnn.

A nearby street light shows the shadow of the big tree outside our window. My eyes burn, but I can't sleep.

Ghghgghnnnn. Mom's snoring is keeping me awake.

The mattress from the pullout coach is on the floor because the metal frame was uncomfortable. I'm two feet from Mom's hospital bed, trying to accustom myself to her snoring by listening for the rhythm.

Ggggghhhh.

My body begins to relax and I allow my dry eyes to close. I cuddle onto my side into a ball and position my pillow to support my neck.

My body flinches, on the verge of sleep, when suddenly I wake fully, realizing something isn't quite right. I sit up. *What is off? What is out of place?*

It's Mom. She has stopped snoring. I don't hear anything. Fumbling out of my covers, tripping off the mattress, I perch over her body. Her mouth is open and her chest barely rises.

I breathe out. *She's alive.*

A warm, subtle, baby-like scent from the oils of her hair and scalp wafts to my nose. Instantly, a smile forms on my face. She smells like Mom. I breathe in the cuddly, human scent of a person at rest—earthy, angelic, grounded, and vibrant. The familiar yet fleeting smell can't be duplicated.

Returning to my mattress, I realize the dilemma. Either she keeps me awake with her snoring, or her silence prevents me from sleeping by igniting my fear that she has died.

CHAPTER 38

Agitation

TODAY MOM HAS BEEN yelling into other dimensions or into her memories. She breaks into sobs every ten minutes. During Jay's lunch break, he helped Mom into the wheelchair so she could enjoy sitting by the open window and smell the fresh fall air. It is the first time she has been out of bed in over a week.

I'm skittish around her, as her angry, unpredictable outbursts catch me off-guard. Mom and Dad never yelled or permitted us to yell in the house when we were growing up. They would physically discipline or use the line "I'm very disappointed in you." The stern tone of voice and hard statement crushed my tender ego. A raised voice was never a part of my everyday world until Alzheimer's struck, wiping away Mom's better judgment and calm conflict resolution skills.

"AaaAaachoo," I sneeze. "Bless you," I say out loud to myself, knowing Mom would say it if she were alert and able.

Comfortable with carrying on both sides of our imagined conversations, I continue with her typical response whenever someone used to say "Bless you" to her. Utilizing the space in the roof of my mouth, I imitate her proper, matter-of-fact, sing-songy reply, "Thank you, He has."

Twisting the corners of my lips into a smirk, I search her countenance, trying to detect recognition. Turning her neck in a slow swivel, she glances at me. After a moment, she permits an enormous smile to permeate her sourpuss face.

✳

The following morning Mom asks, "Did you do it?"

Having no idea what she is talking about, I glance side to side with my hands open and respond, "Did I do what?"

Mom says, "Did I do matches?"

Hesitating, I say, "I am not sure."

"Eree ... matches," she says, sounding sad.

"Do you mean how I am matched up?" I ask.

"Yeah, did you do it? Why didn't you do it?" She continues without my answering. "I watched you. You came out in matches." Tears form in her eyes and she blinks her lids numerous times. "Yeah, you came out in matches. You came out another."

I don't know how to respond without stirring up more anger and upsetting her, so I simply say, "Thank you for taking the time and energy to share this with me." She is putting out tremendous effort to tell me something that I'm not able to translate.

"Oh, same for you. It is good," she tells me and then begins crying. "It is good."

"Do you want a hug?" I offer.

Mom nods, murmuring, "Yeah."

Moving to her, I put my arms on either side of her pillow and upper body, squeezing her inside my forearms. I feel her hot breath through my cotton shirt. Loosening my embrace, I sit at the side of Mom's bed, listening to her incomprehensible ramblings.

"You came out like you. I saw you. NO, you wree ous. You

were supposed. You be down. Trear. I noticed you. You were good. You were good to you. You were no fool. You wre no diss. You were nooo displayed. You will notice my—tears. Its's good. He will notice. How was he? He will know this place. YOU can play. You be good. You. You be goo. Be praying for you. He should be brave. He'll be matches. You be nappin. You be matches. And be good. You be good. You be batches. You be patches. You be batches. He'll be matches. Huh? You be batches."

Mom's talking is louder and more animated. "He is gonna be on your side. He said he is gonna be by soon. He is gonna be on the other side."

I'm not able to calm her, and she is spiraling into anxiety. *Should I leave?* In a soothing voice I ask, "Am I upsetting you?"

"No, it is fine," Mom answers me and then plunges again into her weird tone of voice and garbled words. "BE on your side."

"Are you saying that I need to look out for myself?" I ask.

Mom is peering at me and says in a crystal clear voice, "Yeah. WE are gonna have to. You be batches. Matches be good. I'll help you too."

I interrupt her monologue. "Are you in pain?"

Mom ignores my question. "He'll help him. He'll do down. Down't. He'll be down. He's gonna be down." Mom is sobbing again.

I reach out and hold her hand. *Maybe my challenge is to be in my own essence and love her in the tears.* "Are you scared?"

"NO. He is gonna be down."

"When?"

"I don't know."

"Soon?" I question.

"He will be down. Will he be down. When will he be down?"

I find myself trying to guess if she is talking about death and God coming to greet her. "He will be down when you are ready.

When he comes down, you will be ready," I say, attempting to reassure her.

"Okay."

"You can relax; he will wait till you are ready. There is no hurry."

"What didddid you do?" she asks, raising her eyebrows in my direction.

"It is what I know inside."

"Okay."

"I do know he will wait till you are ready."

"Okay. He is gonna be ... He is gonna do it. He will be by."

"I love you. I will be back later." I feel like my presence is triggering emotion in Mom. I don't know where I will go, maybe to get a cup of tea and write and return when she is less agitated.

"O-kay," Mom says in a quiet voice.

✳

Several nights later, I am sitting next to Mom as orange light spills from the lamp on the dresser, filling the space the sun has abandoned. My eyelids are heavy and my belly is full. Burping a Señor Sam's burrito, I turn the other way so she will not smell the spicy food I had for dinner.

She holds my hand longer than normal and shakes it slightly with each syllable. "Listen to what I say."

I nod obediently, waiting.

She continues in deliberate emphatic speech, "You are good." Then she says, "I want you to have faith."

Is she talking about religion, life, death, love? I don't know how to respond.

"Say yes," Mom says in a zoned-out voice.

CHAPTER 39

Ounces: Five

TIPTOEING UP TO THE frosted glass door at 907 Mary Jane Street, I let myself in and slip off my shoes before walking across the white Berber carpet toward the bedroom. The residents are already in their rooms. I open Mom's door and close it gently behind me. Karen is rocking in the chair that Mom used to rock all of us in as babies. She is reading to Mom in a hushed lullaby voice. I put down my bag and greet each of them. Mom is drifting off to sleep. Karen mouths the words "May I speak with you?" nodding to the huge bathroom.

Karen and I walk into the adjacent bathroom, part of Mom's master bedroom. "Shannon has been giving Mom water. She said you were doing it also. I have tried to wet her lips too, and Mom does seem to want to drink." She states it simply, but I feel confrontation underneath. Shannon is the live-in caregiver at Beth's foster home.

"Uh, I gave her a sip this morning—her mouth was totally dry. I thought we are trying to keep her comfortable." Instantly, I realize I'm wrong. Resigned, I ask, "What has Shannon been doing?"

"She gave Mom about five ounces of water today." Karen's compassionate blue eyes search my face.

"Fuck. Fuck. Fuck. What have I done?" My right hand clamps my mouth while my elbow pushes firmly into my abdomen.

Karen continues, "This is why we took the time to discuss Mom's living will. We all wanted to be on the same page. Mom didn't want to be fed or kept alive, and this included hydration. Does this trigger an emotional component for you?"

Looking down, I say, "No, You're right. I thought it was okay for us to do things to keep her comfortable, but then sips of water spill into drinks and the lines become blurry."

"Are you going to talk to Jay and Dan, or do you want me to tell them?" she asks. "I think they need to know."

My brain feels as if it is going to explode, and my eyes bulge, searching for answers.

Leaning against Dan's kitchen cabinets, my feet slide as the rag rug slips on the red Spanish rock tiles. The tension is palpable, holding the air, which smells of orange peels and freshly split wood, still. I want to crouch down, but I hold my posture with my arms folded tightly in front of me.

"I'm dumbfounded that you didn't understand what we had agreed upon. How many meetings do we have to have?" Dan's voice flambés my skin.

"Dan, I'm sorry. I was wrong. For clarification, it was only about five ounces of water total. I was trying to moisten her lips and keep her comfortable, but then after I left, Shannon started giving her water to drink."

"It isn't the amount that matters, it's the fact that she didn't want to live like this. We had already pushed the envelope of her wishes, and I thought we all agreed that we were ready to follow them. This is why we moved her to the foster home. Are you trying to prolong her inevitable death?" Dan demands. His jaw muscles flex. His words sting my already battered heart from self-inflicted beatings of letting down my siblings and Mom.

"No, I guess I'm not thinking clearly." Then, quieter I say, "Maybe I'm spending too much time there."

He walks to me, still exasperated, and wraps me in a hug as my body trembles. "Kate," he gently says, "this is difficult for all of us."

The aromas of wheat toast and sweet cantaloupe fill the room; my belly rolls. Mom glances at the plate of food, but then looks away. Honoring this living will would be more difficult if she was lusting after food without the ability to eat.

I'm tempted to eat it. *She is not eating anyway, what would it matter?* But on principle, I can't; I can't eat food intended for her and I can't have the staff here believe that she ate it. I need it available on the whim that Mom wants to eat.

I smile gently, remembering Mom's cantaloupe quip that used to be funny until she began repeating it every three minutes. She would offer "Cantaloupe?" holding a fresh, big ripe melon the size of her breast. Then, with a girlish giggle she would answer herself. "Can't elope tonight—Dad's got the car!"

It is two days later. I have been sitting with Mom for two hours. Her cycle is to fall asleep deeply and, within five minutes, wake, startled, lifting her head off the bed—panicked. Sometimes she has a grimace.

I get up and walk to the far side of the bed and sit down in the rocking chair. She appears calm when she sleeps; what is it that is disturbing her? *Here she goes again, yeah, the wide-eyed searching—oh my gosh, it is her tongue; she is choking on her own tongue!* I jump up, wondering what to do. It is obvious from this angle—how did I miss it? I reposition her using all my strength to move her dead weight. I inspect her tongue; it is thick and dry. It must be like Velcro when combined with the bit of moisture expelled from her lungs. I reach toward the sippy cup on instinct. As soon as I feel the rubber grip in my hand, my hand jerks open to drop it. I stop and suddenly question everything I'm doing.

Am I trying to keep her alive? Choking seems like an awful way to die, but she has "Do Not Resuscitate" orders. *I learned CPR and the Heimlich maneuver together; does Mom not want either one? Or does that refer only to food choking?*

I wonder about getting Shannon, the night caregiver. Mom looks at me helplessly and expectantly. I ask, "Do you want me to get Shannon?" Mom motions frantically with her eyes and the slightest shake of her head, while her raspy voice emotes, "Hhhgghyeahh." I jog down the stairs and do everything but go all the way into Shannon's room, knocking, calling, stomping. No response. I hear the footsteps of the elderly resident who lives in the front of the house, and hope I didn't scare her.

Fuck, is this part of honoring her wish? To die choking? Have we decided on this? I don't think I can sit back and watch it happen. I thought I was prepared to be present for a peaceful death but can I be present for an active death?

I return to Mom's room and she is sleeping again. I call Jim, who is a respiratory therapist. He knows about blocked airways. He tells me that rather than increasing the elevation of her whole upper body, I should lift only her head by putting a rolled towel behind her pillow. Then to turn her slightly to one side—that way the tongue will rest in her cheek, rather than covering the airway when it relaxes.

It's so simple. She seems fine now, sleeping a lot and even breathing fourteen times per minute. As far as her living will is concerned, Jim thought it would be okay to reposition to "keep her comfortable."

"LET'S GO NOW." I jolt awake to the drawn-out words of the determined raised voice. I search the dimly lit room. Ah, yes, I'm with Mom. It is only two nights after she was choking in her sleep. I've created a makeshift bed from two shower stools, the rocking chair, a sleeping pad, and a few pillows. It is the same height as Mom's mattress. Lowering her bed rail, I'm able to hold her while we sleep.

"IT'S TIME," she yells. I cuddle close to her.

In a frustrated whine she exclaims, "I'M TRYING." She is breathing fast, about thirty breaths per minute.

I whisper, "I love you."

She doesn't respond, but continues loudly, projecting to the dimensions beyond, "I DON'T KNOW HOW TO."

CHAPTER 40

Hygiene

A YELLOWISH PIECE OF skin is flaking off of Mom's dry, cracked lips. I look closer and see yellow coating building up on her teeth.

Gathering supplies, I remember Aunt Julie teaching me how to clean Mom's teeth with the pink star foam toothpicks.

As I put on small latex gloves I ask, "May I clean your teeth?"

"Sshure," Mom says with a lisp.

At first I try the toothbrush, but her lips are flaccid, and without coordinated control they fall in the path of the brush. I set it aside and reach for an expensive disposable foam star. *Why do these cost so much money?* I dip the star in water, wring it out, and then slide it across her teeth. It doesn't seem to do anything, but I smell the mint from the foam. I turn the star in a circle and it begins to pick up yellow sticky goo from between her teeth. Taking the foam stick out of her mouth, it is already covered and I barely started cleaning. Using a white tissue I dab all sides of the foam, uncovering its original pink. The texture is that of jelly that gums up when it is stuck around the lip of the jar. The color belongs on 1970s tile floor or in a putrid liver. It is jaundice yellow. In the cavity of her cheeks, the yellow is moister, more like thick mucus or egg whites. I have to twirl fast to pick up the coagulating goop. Smelly yeast lingers in her breath and mouth cavity.

The roof of her mouth appears to be rotting; her gums are black and white near her front teeth and have pulled away from her yellowed enamel. When I examine underneath, I see more stickiness caked behind her teeth. After moistening the gums and teeth with the pink star, I reach in with my gloved hand and pull on the gummy bottom edge. A piece the size of a filleted Swedish Fish candy is extracted in a perfect retainer mold of her top teeth. My whole body shivers and I clench my eyes closed. *Whhhho*, I breathe out. It is the grossest thing I have seen or smelled in a long time. And yet, part of me likes feeling successful and productive. Cleaning her teeth gives me something to do that feels useful in a hopeless situation. The bottom "retainer" comes out in smaller sections.

I continue working. Her tongue has a deep gouge in it as if it is cracked, and the yellow crust flakes on her coated tongue. When I put the foam brush back into her mouth, her tongue pushes it out. I put it in again and she begins sucking on the foam before biting down, clamping her jaw tight.

"Open up, let go. Relax your jaw," I say as I attempt to pry the teeth apart with my free hand while shaking the end of the foam stick. Mom's head wiggles like a dog playing tug of war, but she won't loosen her grip.

"Open your mouth lhik dihs," I say while demonstrating a gaping mouth. Her pupils stare at me, and surrounding eye wrinkles pucker into smile lines. Her lips do not move.

Giving up, I hold the stick lightly with one hand so she won't choke on it if she does open her mouth. With the other hand, I begin to delicately peel the yellowish skin off her bottom lip and realize it isn't flesh after all; it is goop from her teeth that stuck to her lip and dried on it like Elmer's glue.

When Mom opens her jaw, I pull out the foam stick, clean it off again, dip it in the water, and then dab off the excess. She has had fillings as long as I can remember. However, it seems her constant consumption of Butter Rums and Diet Pepsi in the last few years has wreaked havoc in her mouth, even with frequent dental appointments. Caramel-colored dots the size of poppy seeds are rotting in her teeth.

Swishing her tongue back and forth in her mouth, she says, "Feels good," in clear words.

Her metal fillings and caps sparkle as I apply a dab of mineral oil inside her mouth to keep the orifice lubricated. Then I put lip cream on her thin, slack lips. *Guunnnp.* Mom is having trouble swallowing the little bit of water and mineral oil that seeped to her throat.

I throw out the pink foam sticks and tissues that are coated in a stale, yeasty beer scent that overpowers the spry mint. Removing the precious gloves as I was taught in lifeguard classes, I attempt to keep the stench of death off my bare skin.

Hearing her belly rumble upon my return to the room, I say, "Oww, Mom, I'm sorry if that bit of water is creating hunger pangs for you."

As I move toward the bed, I realize she is sleeping.

Writing in my journal on the far end of the foldout couch near the marble table, I watch Mom's breathing cycle and the tremors that grip her with a particular breath, causing her whole body to shake. *Was that an emotional release or a side effect of the calming medications?* Other than these tremors, she has been still and quiet all night, which is uncommon. I'm actually taking big breaths again. I hadn't realized it before, but over the past five days, I have been holding my breath around Mom. Every day I'm scared she is going to die.

Curiosity causes me to shake Mom's shoulder. *Is this the stage before death when she becomes unresponsive?*

"Can you wake up?" I ask.

She answers me, "Ye ... uhuh ... yes," with a raspy gremlin voice.

"Can you open your eyes?"

Again Mom replies, "Yeah," lifting her eyebrows, stretching her eyelids. Her eyes remain shut, as if she is looking directly into a bright light in the dark of night.

✳

CHAPTER 41

Love Transcends Borders

MOM USES THE THUMB and pointer finger claw of both hands to pull the material of her nightgown into tiny ant tents. She's aimless, yet persistent at this picking process. Her shrill voice exclaims, "I need you. It is going to be tonight. It is time."

Startled, I drop my book as Mom's agitation breaks the stillness of the evening. Moving to the side of the bed, I wonder if she is talking about death. Taking her fidgety hand in mine, I listen as she continues, "It is tonight. How do I do it? I am afraid." Her gaze searches beyond the colorful *We Love You, Mom* sign that is taped to the ceiling above her bed.

Maybe I could lead her in a meditation? I have no idea how she will feel about it, so I ask, "Mom, may I lead you in a thought process to help calm your anxiety?"

"Shhure," she responds with a small lisp and little emotion, while her pupils continue probing past the white sheetrock overhead.

"Closing your eyes, tune into your body. Notice any sensations that arise," I begin a short introduction. Opening my eye a tiny crack, I notice she has her eyes closed.

During the meditation, whenever I use the word "love" she writhes and moans. I decide to divert from the meditation.

"You can take this love with you. I believe love transcends all borders. Watch as I send love to Dick," I say. I have no idea what it will look like energetically, but figure Mom might see it, since she says she is able to see God.

Softly, I say, "Hello, Dad, I love you. I'm grateful for the role that you play in my life. Thank you for supporting me." My whole body flushes with heat and a smile spreads across my face. There is a thick, perceptible energy around us.

"Love goes from me to the other side and back again. Watch, Mom, I will send you love." Centering my thoughts, I let go of wondering if this is right for Mom. I breathe into my core and send her love. Moving my fingers over the middle of her chest ever so slowly with sensitivity into her aura, I lower my hand. Barely perceptible is the moment when we physically touch and my palm rests delicately on her heart area. Sending her love through my whole body I say, "Thank you for being here and teaching me."

I whisper, "Love crosses all borders. You will be loved wherever you go." A goose-bumped angelic shiver jiggles across my body. I feel honored to be in this tender and vulnerable space with her.

Her heart emits the bass to the musical patter of her swishing blood, billowing lungs, and pulsing energy. The air is electric. Her face is still, her body relaxed. She has fallen asleep.

CHAPTER 42

✳

Rusty Orange

DRESSED IN MY NAVY yoga pants and St. Lawrence sweatshirt, I sit journaling near Mom's bed. Mom is calm. It is noon. Her blood pressure and pulse are high, and her body temperature is normal. Above and below her dry lips, veins creep to the surface. The circles around her eyes are getting darker. Mom's eyes were always a solid, intense sapphire blue surrounding her dark black pupils. Now, her irises are a beautiful clear powder blue.

She had another bowel movement this morning. Its rank smell filled the room and still lingers in the air. Her urine changed from dark yellow to a rusty orange.

It has been two weeks since I first cleaned her mouth. In the last few weeks, her breath has become putrid. It smells as if something died, like an old rat crawled down inside of her, as they do in the walls of homes. Her breath billows in only one direction, forcing the horribly strong concentrated stench of that seething, bloated animal to spill out into the bedroom. It makes sense that because she is dying, there would be different odors, but I had no idea it would smell like roadkill.

When we sleep at night, I crawl into bed next to her, positioning myself away from her wretched breath. I cuddle into her cheek and the side of her neck to avoid the direct line of fire. Usually, she is turned slightly away from me to avoid choking on her own tongue as she sleeps. At full strength, her exhalation makes me gag. Out of the way of her breath, I'm able to stroke her hair.

For the past five years, I have thought this disease was a long death, but these past weeks have been longer than I imagined possible. It's a terrible death—well, not as bad as the vegetative fetal-position alternative. But it does make suicide seem inviting. As crazy as it sounds, suffocation would be better than this, and I half-fantasize about holding a pillow over her … but I can't. I love her too deeply (or maybe not enough).

Mom's new pink flannel nightgown has snaps on the sleeves, similar to children's clothes, to make it easier to dress her. *What would Mom want to wear in her casket? Her rescue squad jacket as a symbol of her contributions and the organization in which she took the most pride? Or maybe her favorite polyester knit baby-blue suit that she has had since I was a kid? What pictures and things should we bring to set up for her memorial service?*

"Come on, let's go," Mom says, her words cutting into my thoughts.

She doesn't appear to be talking to me, so I don't respond.

Mom is dying and yet she is also healing. Her bed sores are getting better—the purple blistery sore that has been on her heel since she was at Chapford looks better. The rest of her skin seems healthier too, as she has fewer dry spots. Even in death there is new life—new cells, hope, and transition.

Mom's saggy skin hangs loose from her bones; the fat that once was stored inside is no longer there. Some fat remains, but not like the bloated 205-pound woman of eight months ago.

Mom's forehead frown and the severe "V" between her eyebrows have softened. I see the outline where the "V" used to be, but it is no longer activated. Additionally, the old sharp-jagged wrinkle in the middle of her brow has been replaced with delicate, graceful rainbow lines that radiate up to her hairline. The rainbow begins and ends at her subtle white eyebrows—each sparkling baby blue is a pot of gold.

CHAPTER 43

Wheelchair Contest

IT IS TUESDAY, ALMOST two years since Dad died. Dan is sitting in the wheelchair in Mom's room, the prized seat. The rest of the chairs are occupied by other family members. Using his arms, he pushes forward and then pulls hard until the front wheels jump off the ground to balance on the rear wheels.

BAM! The front wheels smash down when he loses his balance. He pushes off his toes and is in the air again. His lips disappear inside a firm bite as he concentrates.

Mom stirs lightly.

Knock, Knock.

I answer, "Come in."

"Is everything okay in here?" Beth, a caregiver and the owner of the foster home, peeks inside the door and glances around the room as Dan plunks down the small front wheels.

"Yeah, we're fine. I'm playing around," Dan says.

"I thought I heard a commotion in here," Beth smiles. She walks to Mom, touches her arm lightly, and then leaves the room.

Before she reaches the door, Dan asks, "You want to try?"

She grins, saying, "No, but thanks anyway," and proceeds into the kitchen.

Touching his goatee and rising from the couch, Guy, Karen's husband, says, "Alright, my turn." He grabs Dan's hand, helping him out of the chair. Guy balances with ease, moves forward and back, and then does a full circle to the right and then another circle to the left, before placing all four wheels on the ground again.

Karen exclaims, "What the heck? How did you do that?"

"Uh, it was a lucky first try," Guy laughs and then adds, haughtily shaking his shoulders, "It's my natural athletic prowess."

"No, really, how did you do that?"

"My grandma had a wheelchair when I was kid, and I used to play on it when I'd visit her."

"Then you're disqualified for not disclosing that information sooner. Let me try," Jay says, helping Guy off the chair. Then he adds, "I can beat that."

Within seconds Jay yells, "Uhh. Uhhha—AAAhhhh," as he falls backward in the wheelchair, crashing to the floor.

"You okay?" Karen asks.

The room erupts in laughter. Mom is peacefully lying in her bed, blinking, and in garbled sounds she mutters, "Arrrrurur gura."

Holding Mom's hand, I give her the play-by-play through my laughter. "Jay lost. He fell backwards, but is fine."

"It was me, Mom. I fell," he says, rubbing his calves, still lying on his back in the inverted wheelchair. Jay has a devious, playful smile as he cups his hand toward the door leading to the foster home kitchen and shouts, "Sorry, Mom."

An hour later, Dan, Jay, Karen, and I are the only remaining family members in Mom's room.

"It's going to be sooner than later, but who knows when it'll be. All the arrangements are in place for the funeral home in Oregon to receive the body, do an autopsy, send her brain to NIH, and transport her body to New York. Additionally, we were able to switch to the funeral home in Belleville, instead of the one we used for Dad," Karen says.

"Thanks for doing that," Dan says, "I think I speak for all of us: that's not something I have the energy to tackle right now. But I'm grateful it's done."

"You're welcome," Karen replies, nodding and taking in a breath. Her shoulders are high with stress. "It was a lot of work."

"Even if Mom dies now, can we postpone the funeral for a week to combine it with our trip to NIH for the family study?" Jay asks. "I don't know all the details about when you have to bury a body."

"Once the body is embalmed, it lasts for a long time," Karen says.

I respond, "I'd like to have the funeral right after she dies. This has consumed so much of my life; I'd rather complete everything than bury her in two weeks. Why would you want to wait?"

"Simply put, I hate to fly and don't want to fly twice across the country if I don't have to." Jay's voice is stressed and he aggressively scratches his head.

"Oh, right," I say, seeing the pale angst creep into his face. He has had some awful flight experiences. "In that case I'm fine with waiting."

Suddenly, I stiffen, realizing we are discussing this in front of Mom. I move only my eyes to look at my siblings and capture their attention. Then, I nod toward Mom and grimace.

Dan shrugs and raises his eyebrows.

Karen says, "From what I've read, sometimes it's important for people who are dying to know that everything is being taken care of in preparation for their death." Mom doesn't move. In fact, this is the most relaxed I have seen her all day. She hasn't flinched or seemed offended by our conversation. However, I feel guilty.

✳

It is two days after the wheelchair contest and family funeral conversation. Today is Thanksgiving. It is now seventeen days with no food and little water.

Mom's hands and feet are a dark purple; they are the same temperature as the rest of her body. The flesh is tight to her bones and I can see the veins underneath. Her face still has a nice pinky tone and her lips are reddish-pink. Mom is internal and not responsive. *Is she okay, whatever "okay" means? What time will she pick and why? What day?*

"Mom, I'm going to play football with the family for Thanksgiving. I'll be back later tonight. I want to be with you when you transition, but if you want to be alone, I understand." Mom doesn't move or respond. I kiss her lightly.

Uncle Jim, Dad's brother, is joining us for Thanksgiving. He is the last family member planning to visit. He is cautious, reserved, the classic depiction of a well-mannered priest. He has said prayers with Mom. Depending upon her mental frame of mind, all spiritual bases are now covered, as he is tending to her Catholic upbringing.

The drive is dark and cold to Mary Jane Street where Mom's foster home is located. It is ten o'clock, Thanksgiving night. I've been anxious all day being away from Mom.

I walk up the familiar stairs and let myself in the foster home.

"Hi, Beth," I say. "How's she doing?"

"She's about the same: unresponsive, but peaceful."

Walking with my bag slung over my shoulder, I enter slowly to not disturb her. The lamp behind her is shedding a dim light on the room. I turn up the heat. Putting down my bag, I take off my coat and tiptoe to the side of Mom's bed. Leaning over the bedrails, I touch Mom's arm and say, "Hi, Mom, it's Kate. I love you. I'm back."

"Mom, I'm going to look at your hands," I say.

Moving the blankets, I assess her changes since I was with her this morning. Her delicate, pinkish-white skin on her arms and legs has turned the same scaly, dehydrated purple I witnessed on her hands and feet this morning. Pressing on her ridged fingernail, I watch as it turns white from the pressure and then quickly returns to the ghostly bluish hue. *Is capillary refill determined only if the skin color is normal?* From what I know, her quick capillary refill indicates that death is not imminent, although I have never seen this color of skin outside of a localized bruise.

Her skin has become darker, denser, with less fluid; only veins and bones remain and the thin skin is no longer saggy. Now it is sucked tight to the bones. Further up the arms and legs the skin is loose and scaly where, I presume, her body is taking fluid now.

Figuring how much water is draining from her extremities and how much body mass she has left, I determine that it may be five days for the rest of her body to follow suit in the dense dehydration. But I doubt her organs will continue to function for that long.

"Hughgngnggn." Her breathing is louder and labored. Congestion clogs her throat, making a rattling sound. She makes no attempt to clear the phlegm and appears peaceful except for her breaths. Her right eye is partly open.

A red flush covers Mom's eyebrow area and cheeks. It contrasts with the dark purple-black shadow on her chin and her eyes. A frigid arctic blue tints her nose and mouth. I caress her hairline, moving the white angelic hair completely off her face.

It is eleven p.m. A tingly chime escapes her throat. It sounds like a Tibetan meditation bowl. *What is making that sound?*

Midnight. Mom's breathing has changed again. A high pitched *nnnnn*, like the shaking of a blown light bulb and the other part, *thdthdthdthdthd*, is like a cat purring. I wonder if that is the death rattle that my close friends Shady and Lucinda described to me. The purple color has moved even further up her body. *Is this the mottling that the hospice booklet* Gone From My Sight *describes in the stages of death?* I cuddle Mom, nuzzling behind her ear, smelling her subtle, lightly salty scent. My eyelids are heavy. *Should I call my siblings? Am I crying wolf?* Having listened to her new breathing changes and calculated it so many times before, I simply notice it and struggle to stay awake. I want to be alert if she dies tonight.

I proceed to fall into the deepest sleep of my life.

CHAPTER 44

Upside-Down Goodbyes

SLEEPING INCHES FROM MOM'S body, I wake to Beth's strong hands tenderly touching the chilled flesh of Mom's face. Using my index fingers, I remove the crusty goop from the corners of my eyes and blink through the hazy fog of my vision. Mom's lips and skin around her eyes are ghost-blue. Morning light filters into the window; checking the clock, I see it is 8:45. *How did I sleep so soundly? I had wanted to monitor her throughout the night. Did I have any significant dreams?*

Mom's breathing, quick and shallow, still has the purring chime quality. However, now her nostrils flare with each breath.

Stethoscope and thermometer in hand, Beth's firm hand moves to Mom's chest and follows the desperate concaved rise and fall. I reach for my glasses so I can see every detail of Beth's wise countenance. Her face is serene on the surface, though concern is rippling beneath her tight eye muscles.

"She will tire herself out breathing like that."

My eyes pop open. "How long do you think?" I tentatively ask, knowing how most medical personnel avoid estimating the time remaining.

"If this continues, it will be today," she says.

Panic rises inside of me. I don't say anything out loud, but inside I'm thinking, *What? Today? Today?*

"I'm not going to change her this morning; I don't want to disturb her," Beth says.

Beth silently leaves the room and I hold Mom in a tight hug.

"Good morning, Beautiful. I love you," I whisper.

I watch the striped, feathery clouds turn the light-blue sky tangerine and fuchsia. Entranced, I watch the outstanding brilliance dawdle across the picture window. The sky perfectly matches the Gerber daisies on Mom's bed tray; orange is her favorite color.

Beth taps lightly on the door. "I think your siblings should be notified. Should I call them?"

"No, I will." I glance at the clock. *Yikes, I have been watching the sky for an hour.*

Jay arrives right away with his kids. He is teary and serious. We set up a *Barney* video for Jake and Grace in their makeshift playroom, the huge walk-in closet.

A half hour later, Karen arrives. Her face is red and swollen, and her voice is tight and intermittently screechy. "I called the relatives to tell them the latest," she says, and as she moves toward Mom, her jaw begins to shake. "Mom, we are here with you in this time." Karen's eyes jump from Mom's face to her gasping chest. As she surveys Mom's developments, her brows furrow and her lips form a thin line. Her eyes tense.

I move the blankets so Karen can see the mottling on Mom's arms. Reaching out a supple hand, Karen delicately touches Mom's limb. Her pale pink skin contrasts with Mom's purple and navy splotches, making it appear even more grotesque.

Karen lets out a whimper, "Hhuuow," as the corners of her mouth curve downward and she swiftly covers it with a cupped hand.

Lori, who was at her school diligently preparing lesson plans, stops in to pick up Grace and Jake. She begins crying also.

I feel immune to the instant grief my family is experiencing as they enter the room. I guess because I have been with Mom through the overnight decline, it isn't a shock to me. If anything, I'm feeling comforted having my family here with me.

Mom seems calm, unaffected by any of us.

As Lori is getting ready to leave with the kids, Jay squats down to their level. He says, "You know Grammie is dying? She will probably die today and you will not see her again."

They peer over at Mom and nod. Mom is like a toy that they used to play with and crawl over, but for months she has been broken and her batteries have worn out—she doesn't laugh or run or hold them anymore.

"Do you want to say goodbye to Grammie?" Jay asks, scooping them up, one on each side, supported by his strong arms. They dangle their arms around his neck.

They glance at Mom, shaking their heads side to side, no. They turn toward Jay and begin to play with him, plugging his nose and trying to tickle his armpits. Unable to hold their wiggling bodies, he sets them down on the rug. "You can't catch me," Grace says playfully as she scampers to the door where Lori is waiting.

Jake is still holding onto Jay's nose. Flipping Jake up in the air, Jay inverts him, his blonde hair hanging an inch off his scalp. Jay asks, "What about an upside-down goodbye?"

A little giggle is heard. "Goodbye, Grammie."

"My turn," Grace says, running to Jay's side.

Jay sets Jake down and lifts Grace while holding her waist. Her knees bend over his shoulders, and her brown hair brushes the quilt on Mom's bed.

Laughing and waving she says, "Bye, Grammie."

"Do any of you need time alone with Mom?" I inquire. Karen and Jay indicate it is not important at this time.

Jay lifts Mom's shoulder and proceeds to envelop her in his arms. With his head near hers, he sings "Amazing Grace" in his deep, full voice. The familiar song, and his affection for Mom, brings a quiver to my throat; I'm only able to hum through my trembling vocal cords. Karen harmonizes between her tears, "We've no less days to sing God's praise, than when we first begun." The cathedral echo of their voices fill the room. Karen, in an overly serious voice, sings a final "Ahhh-Meennnn," with a tiny playful smirk scarcely visible under her wet cheeks.

During the song, Mom's breathing changes. The air is thick and lacking adequate oxygen for me to breathe with ease. I feel a flush over my heart and a sensation hover over my scalp. The roots of my hair tingle and a shiver slithers down my body. *It feels like Dad.*

Jay's red eyelids are moist. He clutches her shoulders in his tanned, solid grip and says, "I love you Mom … fffsssssshhhh," he sniffs, "I love you." Lowering his head, he moves away. He crawls under my fuzzy velour blanket on the couch to begin the long wait.

Karen and I glance at each other and at Mom in her flowered flannel nightgown. I move my arm underneath Mom and rest my right hand on the center of her chest. Karen holds Mom's left hand while stroking her wrist and forearm.

Mom's breathing stops. Karen glances at the second hand on her watch. Thirty seconds go by. *Was that her last breath?* I freeze. Mom breathes again. I whisper, "Jay." He doesn't hear me. Louder, I say "Jay." Seeing my nod, he returns to the bed. By Jay wrapping his arm over Mom, she becomes encased in a full hug between our arms. I take her right hand in mine.

In clear, steady words, Karen says, "We will be fine; you can go when you want. We love you. It is okay to go. We will be okay and you will be okay."

Suddenly, I remember that Dad used to say: "Maureen will know that she is loved—no matter how deteriorated her mind becomes, she will know our special handshake. Even on her death bed, she will know I love her." Holding Mom's hand in mine, I give her the special shake. I continue the handshake every minute or so.

Jay says, "I'm sorry I got mad at you when you tried to make me eat my peas as a kid. And I'm sorry for being such a pain in the butt. Thanks for always playing with me and helping me. I love you, Mom. Lori, Grace, and Jake love you. You led a good life and are a good person. Your heart is kind and generous."

Mom's breathing is continuing to slow. She has stopped taking in air again. We wait in silence and Karen squints at her watch. Then Mom opens her lungs again, as if she never stopped.

I clear my throat. "Thanks for letting me be part of this process. May your way be blessed. May your heart be well. On the other side souls will greet you. You are loved." I complete my words with the coded handshake.

Then Karen says, "Dick loves and supports you. Dan loves and supports you. Bob loves and supports you. Todd loves and supports you ..." she continues the pattern, listing off individuals from our family, Mom's family, and Mom's friends.

Mom stops breathing again and then she grasps my hand in a tight squeeze. The rest of her physical body remains static and peaceful. Her strength surprises me, coming from such a feeble body. Her hand releases and then contracts again multiple times before letting go of both my hand and life as we know it. I continue rubbing her hand with my thumb and squeezing the coded handshake. My lips press together as I suck them tight to my teeth, filling in the gaps. Heavy marble tears drop onto the bed sheet.

CHAPTER 45

Warm Body

BETH ENTERS THE ROOM with reverence and even-tempered acceptance of a life passed on. She seems accustomed to death. She reaches to close Mom's dark half-opened eye. *I know she is dead; her eyelids don't need to be closed for me. Why is she doing this—for her own comfort?* The eye closes most of the way, but remains open a crack. Then, Beth moves Mom's legs together and folds her arms over her abdomen, placing her hands on top of one another.

"Why are you doing that?" I ask.

"Rigor mortis is already setting in. When a body hardens in one position, it is very hard to reposition it."

I always thought people were simply scared of the empty pupils staring at them. The thought to push the lids closed manually didn't occur to me, although I have seen countless movies and TV shows wherein death is signified by hidden eyes, disappearing pupils.

What does occur to me is that I'm not the least bit terrified of the eyes or her dead body; it seems normal. *Why is our society sanitized from this process? I'm so curious about everything and wonder how long until I follow her in death. What will it feel like?*

I spend a long time holding her dead body. My touch gradually moves to her core, following the warmth as it dissipates out of the body. I can feel vibration within it.

The body's midsection gurgles and sputters deep in her bowels. *What is the swirling energy under my hands? Is her soul hovering near? When does death officially occur by medical calculations and by our soul experience? Is it the same time? Was the last breath the same as the last heartbeat?* Her heart seems to beat for a half hour after her breathing stops; however, I know my perception of time is off, and I believe that is scientifically impossible. *Is this how some people in the olden days got buried alive, because of the opposing signs of life and death in the body?*

I tell my siblings what I feel. They gape at me skeptically and have no desire to experience it. They are done spending time with Mom's body. Before they leave Mom's room, we discuss funeral arrangements and when to clean out the huge metal barn that we have used for Mom's storage.

I'm transfixed by the process of dying. Maybe I will go to the mortuary with her body and watch everything that they do to prepare the body, and view the autopsy. *Will I be able to see the plaque that has overtaken her brain with my bare eye?*

Karen asks in a concerned tone, "Do you want someone to come in here and make an actual declaration that she is dead?"

"No, I don't need that. I know she is dead, but I don't understand what I'm feeling." *Am I crazy? Does anyone else spend a couple of hours with a dead relative?*

Karen continues, "If I ask the funeral home to come pick her up in an hour, does that give you enough time with her body? I'm aware that we need to get an autopsy done within a certain time frame for her harvested brain to be useful to NIH's research on Alzheimer's disease. Also, the earlier they get her body, the more likely they will be able to use some of her organs for donation.

However, her body may be too depleted from lack of food and liquid to be useful to anyone else."

"Yes, I'm fine—an hour is fine," I say. I'm too tired to travel with her body. I need to rest. The autopsy will provide the final confirmation and official diagnosis of Alzheimer's. I have yet to fill out the information to be sure my brain also goes to NIH when I die to become part of the collection. *Will my brain go on a shelf next to Mom's?*

CHAPTER 46

Charades

MOM DIED FOUR HOURS ago.

Restless energy and not knowing when we would all be together again pushed us to the barn and to the business of cleaning up, consolidating, dividing, donating, and throwing out.

"Does anyone want numerous pairs of ancient cross-country skis that have been in our possession for twenty years?" There is a moment's hesitation as Dan asks, wearily looking up to the second level of the barn where the rest of us are sorting and organizing Mom and Dad's stored belongings. Dan and Jim are loading the trailer bound for Goodwill.

Jay yells, "Hey, they probably paid five dollars for those skis at Salvation Army." Then, with the next breath he says, "Pitch them."

"A box of Christmas tins? Mismatched plastic containers?" Jay asks.

In unison the rest of us respond, "Pitch 'em!"

Jay drops the boxes from the second floor to the first, scattering the contents. Dan jumps out of the way to avoid getting hit by the boxes. Black widows that line the edge of the barn scurry to their spiral-spun homes.

Dan shouts, "You want this job? I will switch places with you and hurl things in your direction and let you clean it up." He leans down to pick up the remnants from the dropped boxes to chuck them at Jay.

Dodging tin lid Frisbees, Jay yells, "I'm sorry. Okay."

They both take a swig from their beers.

A couple hours later, I'm exhausted. "I'm done. I have a headache, I'm dizzy, and don't have energy to continue."

"Okay, just another half an hour—we are almost done," one person counteroffers. This person wants to throw everything away and I don't want to make hasty decisions.

"You can keep going if you want, but I'm done," I state firmly. Never am I this assertive; I usually give in to accommodate others, but I have nothing left. My pile of Mom and Dad's things is growing along with my headache and sadness.

That evening after dinner, we sit in Dan's living room, some of us on the black leather furniture, and some of us on the floor. We are reminiscing about Mom and her crazy antics.

Jay laughs as he begins speaking. "My kids and I were at the playground with Mom. I told her it was time to go. I had Jake in my arms and was holding Grace's hand and we were walking toward the car. I heard Mom say, 'I gotcha, let's go.' She had picked up a blonde-haired boy who was the same age as Jake, and was following me to the vehicle. I said, 'Put that boy down, it isn't Jake.' Mom looks at the squirming boy, then at the Jake in my arms, and said 'Oops,' and puts him on the playground. I was scared the police were going to come after us for attempted kidnapping.

"Another time at the playground, Mom fell down and was screaming for help saying, 'My legs are broken. I need an ambulance.' I knew it was a minor scrape, but she wouldn't be convinced."

Jay stands up and begins acting out the scene. "I tried lifting her up with my hands under her armpits. At that height, she should have been able to tuck her legs underneath and stand up, but she held her legs out perpendicular. I told her, 'Mom, put your legs down.' But she replied, 'They are broken.' By this time, people are staring at us. I put her back on the ground, and finally get her to crawl toward the slide by crawling along beside her." Jay is crawling across the floor with imaginary Mom. "Then, she manages to stand while holding onto the slide, at which point she forgets about her 'broken' legs and trots off to play again."

We are all cracking up laughing when we hear *Ddddad, Ddddat*. It is Dan's cell phone. He walks into the kitchen. "Shhh," he says, slicing his right hand quickly through the air, silencing all sound and movement.

"Yes, so someone called you about Mom?" More silence. "Uhhu." I watch him through the wide opening that forms the kitchen counter and the living room bar. His face is strained, white.

Mom is dead—what can be the stressor now?

I figure it is a relative who found out about Mom, and is calling to touch base with us. We are quiet, listening for clues as to whom it might be.

"I'm so sorry. Is there anything that I can do? Do you want me to notify anyone for you?" He pauses, a pen and paper in hand. Then, staring at us, he says, "Yes, they are here with me. I will tell them. One of us will call you soon."

Gradually, he pulls the phone away from his ear.

"Kathi died."

"Kathi?" a voice asks.

"Aunt Kathi," Dan clarifies. "That was our cousin Julie. Their family was with her this morning in the hospital, and then she took a quick downward turn. It sounds like maybe pneumonia, some sort of cancer complication."

No one moves or even breathes. Even the fire in the nearby fireplace falls silent, or maybe my ears have stopped listening. Cold chills eerily grab at my shoulders.

"Holy shit," breaks the silence.

"Mom's death was expected. Kathi's death wasn't. It doesn't seem fair," says another voice.

"How are they doing?"

"Still in shock," Dan replies.

Dan's face hasn't broken from the rigid, somber intensity. "They're flexible about when to have Kathi's memorial service, but we need to figure out whose service to have first and then allow enough time for the relatives to travel between New York and North Carolina to make the second funeral. Karen, do you still have the NIH information with you about how to do the autopsy? Julie needs it so Kathi's brain can be sent for research too."

"Yeah, I'll grab it from the car."

"Okay," Dan says. Turning to the sink, he takes a shiny silver pot and scrubs away dinner's debris. His strong, broad shoulders hunch forward.

Were they spiritually linked, both being strong Christians? Mom died at 11:30 a.m. Pacific Time and Kathi died at 11:30 p.m. Eastern Time—nine hours apart.

How do we deal with two deaths in the family in one day?

CHAPTER 47

Ten Books

MOM DIED THREE MONTHS ago. Wind is pounding the side of our double-wide trailer, rocking it on its foundation. Rain pings off the tin siding. I'm reading my hospice volunteer manual when Jim arrives home from work.

"Look at you. You are always sad," Jim says. I'm sitting on the floor; he takes a seat near me on the couch. He holds his palms open, before clasping them together. The tone of his message is strong, but his voice quivers. "It's like you don't even want to be happy. I can't make you smile anymore. No matter what I do, you don't laugh."

I hurriedly pick up the wadded tissues that are strewn over the carpet as I say, "I'm processing a lot since Mom and Dad died." Now that I'm relieved of Mom's dependency, the reality that I could get Alzheimer's and the opportunity to find out continually occupies my thoughts. I pull my knees up tight to my chest and wrap my arms around them. "I'm sad, you are right, but it doesn't feel out of proportion with the reality of my life."

"It might not be out of proportion, but look around you," he says, spreading both arms and pointing to the table, walls, and floor. "You have ten books on death and dying that you are actively reading." His voice cracks and tears well up in his eyes. "You are going to hospice training. You have pictures of your parents all around. It's like you have created a memorial of sorts, and there is no room for new life." Over his right shoulder, Dad and Mom stare down at me from their graduation and engagement photographs.

My face blazes hot and my teeth clench as I listen to his words. *I am not depressed. I'm feeling my emotions. That is healthy.*

Heavy teardrops are erased from both of his eyes with the pads of his right fingers. He continues to look at me. I know how much he hates to cry. *Am I totally off balance? Is there truth to what he is saying?*

Timidly, I glance around the familiar living room with fresh sight, changed now by his perspective and the honesty of his tears. There is a stack of books about death on the table, and another four in the bedroom. My hospice volunteer manual lies open on the floor. *Tibetan Wisdom for Living and Dying* audiotapes are under my car keys and sunglasses. Every wall is covered with pictures of my parents, sayings about death, or letters they had written to each other or me. I use their vehicle, living room furniture, dishes, table, chairs, towels, sheets, and even the duct-taped Rainbow vacuum. It is as if I'm keeping them alive, but by doing so, the memories, like a vampire, are sucking out my life.

Tears fall from my eyes now. "I don't know how to go on with my life. I miss their belief in me." My heart is beating fast and my voice is a whisper. "Why live if I have the gene? What is the point?"

"I don't know, Kate, but there is no sense wasting your life too." He sits down next to me on the floor and leans against the plaid foam-cushioned couch—the same couch Mom sat on when we watched *Do You Remember Love?* He puts his arms around me.

"I can't support you any more than I already am. I want to be happy, but I can't be happy with you always sad."

A couple weeks later, Jim stands in front of me in the living room. We haven't spent much time together since our last conversation. He's been working out of town. I rock slowly in the rocking chair. He states, "I'm going to apply for a teaching job in New York. The cost of living is high here and I hate my job. I want to teach, and there are no health education positions in Oregon. You're welcome to come with me—I miss that area and my family." Jim's arms are crossed in front of him and his left hand rests on his right ribs. His lungs make a hollow, thumping sound when he taps on them with a cupped hand.

He has been talking about this for awhile. He hasn't asked me, but he is ready to be married after ten years together, and he wants kids. I'm scared of marriage, kids, commitment; I have to know my gene status first.

I asked Jim to go with me to NIH in Maryland to find out my genetic status, but he has been busy with work. He can't afford the time off because he was absent for a week when Mom died. Maybe it is best I wait to find out my status if he is leaving; one emotional trauma at a time is enough. I thought he would be my support person, but at this point that wouldn't be the best choice. The support person is supposed to be someone who will be in your life for a long time. I have no idea what the future holds for Jim and me.

My heart is shutting down from desperation and grief. I feel resigned to the inevitable. "I will miss you if you go. I don't want you to leave, but I understand. I can't see myself in upstate New

York. It holds too many memories of Mom and Dad and besides it is conservative—I would feel boxed in there." Then, trying to claim some control, I say, "I need to explore more of who I am at a core level and date other people." *How can I know if I want to marry him if I haven't dated anyone else?*

I drop my head between my hands, my fingers outstretched, and tears fall in my lap. He's my high school sweetheart. Everything I do, I would rather do with him. We love each other, enjoy each other's family—I thought we would get married and grow old together.

I stand, take his hand, and lead him to the couch where we fall together, crying.

Four months later, Jim does move and we end our relationship. With newly engraved parental headstones behind me and my unknown genetic status ahead of me, I won't allow the vows "till death do us part."

I saw my reflection in Mom's eyes—a liability even without any clinical symptoms. If I become ill, there will be no control of this desperate need for companionship, distraction, and reliance that already resides within me. In my mind, Mom's disease killed Dad. I feel a moral obligation to ensure that another person does not die because of me. My father's death was a huge disservice to this world. I can't imagine enslaving another to my possible future.

Two birds with one stone, as they say.
But I will keep others at bay,
Making it one for one my way.

CHAPTER 48

Cheek Swabbing

A WHITE VAN WITH the purple and orange FedEx logo zooms up my driveway. A man jumps out, handing me an envelope, and asks for my signature. The summer sun blazes down on the wooden deck. Jim moved nearly a year ago; my car is the only one in the driveway.

Walking to the trailer house door, I notice the return address is NIH and I begin to squish the uneven bulges inside the large envelope. Pulling on the tab, I open the cardboard overnight/special delivery package. Goosebumps pop up on every inch of my body as I peer inside, finding the cheek swabbing kit. *Whoa, this process of finding out my genetic status is faster than I even imagined. Am I ready for this?*

I pull out the contents, spreading them on the floor in front of me, reading each and every word of the directions twice. *Is this the dam that is holding back all my potential? Once it breaks, will I be free either way?*

It is the following morning and my mouth is dry and tastes horrible—morning breath, thick and stagnant. I'm not allowed to drink water or brush my teeth.

236

The anonymous labeling stickers are on the test tube vials, and the white pipe cleaners sit in front of me. Sick to my stomach, I take the plastic tube in my hand, open my mouth, and rub the bristles around three times on my inner cheek. Putting the tube into the vial, tears brim up.

One cheek swabbed, one to go. My stomach pulls tight; I feel ready to dry heave. *If I'm this emotional now, how will I do finding out?* Twirling the other brush inside my left cheek, I hope I'm doing this correctly.

Cutting the stem of the cell brush collector, I also cut the umbilical cord to my previous way of life and all that sustained me. *What will keep me alive? Will I want to stay alive to be a case study for Alzheimer's disease?* Realistically, either I have the gene or I don't, and the only thing changing is my knowledge of it.

I can't stop weeping as I sit here alone.

CHAPTER 49

Divulgence

WATER SWIRLS OFF THE paddle, creating liquid tornadoes with each stroke. I'm in front and Andy's in the back of the canoe. We paddle in unison, moving smooth and swift to explore the swampy inlet of Emigrant Lake. Andy and I met six weeks ago, when he came to town to mountain bike with friends. Since then, we have seen each other numerous times even though he works near San Francisco doing marine construction. Despite my resistance, I have already fallen in love.

"There is something I've been wanting to tell you," I begin. "My heart already knows the answer to this next question, but my brain needs to hear your reply. This information is confidential and only my family and a few close friends know it. Are you willing not to share it with anyone, even if we end up hating each other someday? I know that is highly unlikely, but I have to ask for my own peace of mind."

I turn halfway around so I can see him. Andy's brilliant azure eyes are steady under his sandy brown eyebrows and smooth, shaved scalp. He stops paddling to answer. "You asked me the other day what qualities I like most about myself and I told you that you can trust me, even with your heart. I'm good at keeping secrets and I will not say anything to anyone," Andy's clear voice answers without hesitation.

"Ahhhhhha." I exhale this sound in a massive breath from every cell in my body, one I have been holding for a month. He wins my heart every time he talks or looks at me. "Thank you."

We glide silently through the lily pads in the green canoe, pausing to listen to the chorus of birds in the nearby brush. The blue jay is the only distinguishable squawk to my unlearned ear. *How do I begin? Do I start with the recent cheek swabbing or the history?*

"I told you my mom died of Alzheimer's disease. I haven't told you that my grandmother and her twin sister died from complications related to Alzheimer's. My aunt and uncle also have early-onset Alzheimer's disease. My aunt is in a care facility. My uncle is showing symptoms, but he still works independently and lives at home."

Nervously, I look over my right shoulder. My weight shifts the canoe, rocking it side to side. Andy pushes two fingers behind his right earlobe and tilts his head to the side. Straining to hear my every word, he waits for me to continue.

"Well, the other part of the story, you may have guessed by now, is that it is genetic and I have a fifty percent chance that I also carry that same gene." I move my head as if looking at the scenery, but I'm not taking it in. My mind is busy processing what I will say next and wondering how he will respond.

"Why don't you stop paddling and turn around so I can look at your face while you talk to me," Andy softly proposes.

I bite the inside of my cheek, debating with my inner feminist about letting him do all the work for me. Slowly, I take my paddle out of the water and watch the separation as crystal water dribbles off the smooth wood and into Emigrant Lake. I rest the paddle across the gunnels. My fingers hang loose as my thumbs touch the flesh where tender calluses are forming.

I keep looking forward.

"This is my biggest stress. It occupies so many of my thoughts and choices about life. You have been asking where I see myself long into the future, but I don't have any long-term goals." I straddle the seat, so I can look easily at him, but don't turn fully toward him. He is paddling purposefully with ease and grace. The skin is tight on his round, fit face, permitting me to see that the bones and muscles underneath are serene.

He says, "I notice whenever we talk about the future, the tone of our conversations changes and either you quickly switch the subject, or you get off the phone. I was wondering what was going on and I'm glad you waited to tell me in person. You are a remarkable person to have so much weighing on you, and still you are amazing."

I feel the compliment flush my face with heat and I turn away. *What does he see?*

"I need to find out my status," I say. "I'm in the process of doing that now. If I don't have the gene, I have no idea what my life will be like. If I have the gene, I will never get married or be in a long-term relationship again. It is too much of a burden to put on anyone."

Intently listening, he slowly answers, "I knew some of this, but hadn't realized the extent to which it affects your life. It is something a 28-year-old woman shouldn't have to think about," he shrugs his shoulder, "but that is also the way life comes."

He moves the life vests to the center of the canoe and gives me a "come here" motion with the open cup of his hand. The canoe is steady as his body moves gracefully to the center. Kneeling on a life vest with his back resting on the cross support, he holds open his arms to me. I look around the lake—he has paddled to the middle and there are no obstacles in sight. I shimmy toward him, trying not to rock the boat. As soon as his hands touch my arms, I melt fully into his muscular chest, sobbing.

Looking out over his bicep, I see an osprey spiraling in the distance. Andy loosens his grip, lightly kisses my forehead, and slides a wisp of hair out of my face.

"I don't completely get it, but I'm beginning to understand the impact that this has on your life. Thank you for trusting me." Then he challenges, "I'm puzzled when you say that when you find out your status, if you have the gene, you will push people away. Kate, why do you protect those around you? What if someone actually wants to be there for you and wants to enjoy the years you do have left? What if it is worth it to someone else? Pushing people away isn't giving them a chance to make up their own minds and enjoy some time with you."

I notice my mouth is slightly open, surprised he is questioning me. *How naïve. He hasn't been through it, so he doesn't know how terrible this disease really is.* But his questioning catches me off-guard, so I respond, "Yeah, I guess not. I don't have any big answers—I will think about it. I'm pretty stubborn."

On his return trip to San Francisco, Andy calls. "Thanks for making me so happy. I can't go through life la-de-da with you— you make me think and I like that."

I'm in my living room, perched on a chair, smiling. "Thanks for saying that. I often feel like I'm beyond intense for other people. Andy, if I have the gene and freak out and push everyone and you away, can you still not tell anyone why I disappeared?"

"You won't be the first woman who never wants to speak to me again," he replies, comfortable protecting my intense secret. "I know that when you find out, the news will be so big that if you have the gene or if you don't, you may push me away with either outcome."

My heart jumps and cold chills spread up my neck and into my ears.

He continues, "So give me direction—what do I do? Give you the space because you ask and I respect you? Or stay near because I want to and I think on some level you want me to?"

I'm speechless. My heart silently chants, *Stay. Stay. Stay,* while my head instructs, *Run away now. Too serious already. Run. Run. Run.*

Returning home the next evening from bartending at the Oregon Shakespeare Festival, I have a message from Andy. I drop my mail on the couch and excitedly punch in my calling card number and then his phone number.

His groggy and deeper-than-normal voice answers.

"Hi, Andy," I hesitate, hearing his voice. "Do you want me to call you tomorrow so you can get some sleep?" He stayed with me the night before until eleven p.m. and then drove through the night to San Francisco, arriving an hour before work started this morning.

"No, I want to talk with you. I stopped by Borders tonight and bought a book about Alzheimer's. I wanted to get *Decoding Darkness,* the book that features your family, but they didn't have it, so I ordered it online. I bought *The Forgetting* by David Shenk. Have you heard of it?"

"No, I haven't. I would love to look at it and see its approach to Alzheimer's. I haven't found a really good book about the emotional impact of Alzheimer's disease."

"Maybe that is for you to write," Andy says casually.

Gulp—I haven't told him that I want to write about it. I pause for a moment, gathering my thoughts. "I think that is a big piece for me."

"You should do it," he says without hesitation. He continues, "When I came home, I looked up the Memory Ride on the Internet and saw a picture of you with a huge smile, hugging another person. I also researched information about Alzheimer's on the website for NIH. Then, I found a cheap flight to Bethesda, Maryland. I know I'm not a likely candidate, but I would go with you, if you want me to, when you decide to find out your genetic status."

"Wow, thanks for the offer. I think you must be crazy. Holy shit! I can't believe you did all of that. Why?"

"I want to understand where you are coming from," he calmly replies.

Why, Andy? Why immerse yourself so fast in all of this? Why do you like me so much? I feel honored, afraid, and like I need to hurry and push you away before it is too late. Are you trying to be sure you have an "in" with me if I push everyone else away? Quit being so nice to me—it's uncomfortable and I don't know how to handle it.

CHAPTER 50

*

Rude Questions

COOLING OFF DURING A coed soccer tournament in Ashland, a month after Andy's surprise offer to travel with me to Maryland, I plop down, exhausted, along with other players from all different teams to watch the championship game. Flushed, I guzzle water to rehydrate my body.

Taking off my cleats and socks, I pull back the grass-stained shin guards. Beads of sweat lay underneath.

Suddenly, I hear a man's voice behind me. "Hey, I see on the roster that you're a Preskenis. Are you related to the other Preskenises in town?" I barely know him, but recognize that he works with one of my siblings. He is seated under a white portable shelter ten feet from me.

"Yes," I say smiling, proud of our amiable reputation.

His next question emotionally slide-tackles me, leaving me speechless.

"Do you know your genetic status?"

What?

First shock, then fear, and finally anger rips through every muscle in my body that was relaxing. I'm now in fight-or-flight status. As if sizing up the opponents, I glance around and quickly count fifteen people within earshot.

Cringing, I turn toward the game. Rubbing my shins with my hands, dirt and grass mix with sweat droplets. I take another sip of water. It burns my throat going down.

"Phew, man, that's a hard decision and not one easily answered," I finally say, sidestepping the question. Reaching for my toes, I begin to massage them as I pretend to intently watch the game in front of me, all the while covertly planning my escape.

How did that secret follow me to the field? I find myself curling my toes under and gripping them hard with my fingers.

I realize it isn't completely his fault. As technology advances, society at large does not know the appropriate social graces or sensitivity that need to accompany this uncharted and fascinating territory of genetic awareness. Still, I want to fire inappropriate questions back at him. My mind creates all kinds of hypothetical scenarios and accompanying questions that are socially taboo: *Do you have AIDS? Are you cheating on your wife? Are you taking Viagra? Is your 15-year-old daughter pregnant? Have you ever claimed bankruptcy? Do you like anal sex? Are you snorting cocaine?*

✳

CHAPTER 51

The Least of Worries

BRIGHT YELLOW, ORANGE, AND blue flames dance in the brick fireplace of the beach cabin that belongs to Andy's grandmother. Shadowy details of the family name engraved in the handmade grate crafted by Andy's uncle become visible. Four generations ago, the first family members settled near the Columbia River. The air has a hint of canvas camp smell. It is early evening and the sun has already set into the ocean off Long Beach. Behind the living room's green and white vertical-striped curtains, darkness settles on the breezy fall night.

"You don't have allergies, do you?" Ann, Andy's mom, quizzes me. She is seated in an upholstered armchair with dark, wooden arms. I'm standing near the fire to shake the chill of the evening. Andy is on a torn sage ottoman between Ann and me. We have pulled the chairs and ottoman into a semicircle around our source of heat.

"Uh, not really, until I shift to a new environment. I had them in Kentuc—"

"I mean, you weren't a sickly kid, were you?"

I shake my head side to side, wondering if she is looking for flaws and if she already suspects Alzheimer's. A cold twinge brings my shoulders up.

"I mean, you don't look like you were a sickly kid—you look so healthy." She continues talking on the inhale, her hazel eyes shining in the firelight.

"I know allergies are awful for kids to have." She looks proudly at Andy. "Andy never had any, and my mom always said to try and breed them out. My youngest daughter, now, she had allergies all her life. She sure tried hard, but she always had to struggle so much more than the other kids."

Andy pipes up. "Yeah, but look at her now, she's a lawyer." He crouches, poking the logs and playing with the damper, casting a dark silhouette on the far wall.

Ralph, Andy's dad, is sitting in his chair, engaged, but quiet. He glances up at me and then to Ann before returning his gaze to the flickering light. Ashen wood smoke mixed with crisp autumn air waft into the house when the wind blows down the chimney.

Ann resumes her questioning. "So now, Andy mentioned your mom and dad have passed away. What happened to them? How long ago did it happen? I don't mean to pry, but how old were you? What an awful thing to lose your parents." Her voice rests as she sips from an orange can of Live Wire Mountain Dew. *We both like Mountain Dew; at least we have one thing in common.*

I touch the stone hearth, surprised it's so cold near the blazing fire. Staring into the flames, I slowly say, "My father died of a heart attack four years ago and my mother had Alzheimer's disease and passed away two years ago." Before I gather my next sentence, she interrupts my thoughts.

"How old were your parents? They must have been young."

"Dad was 55 and Mom was 58."

"Alzheimer's at such a young age? I haven't heard of it that young. How did they diagnosis it or even recognize it?"

"It's called early-onset when it hits someone that young," I say as I clear my throat. I hate not knowing what she will ask next.

"How awful, but you have siblings, right? Are you close to them?"

"Yes, I am close to them; we've been through a lot together."

"How many siblings do you have and where do they live?"

"I have five siblings; one sister and four brothers."

"Six of you, whoa, that is a lot for one family. We have a lot also, but that was due to a previous marriage," she says almost under her breath. Then, louder, and without taking a break, she continues. "Now, were your parents Catholic, or did they simply like children?" she says with a giggle and a grin. Her fingernails fluff the reddish-brown hairline at her forehead. Firelight glitters off Ralph's balding scalp and his broad frame squarely fills the chair in which he sits. Leaning forward, his logger's hands massage his newly constructed knee.

I let my shoulders drop. "The four of us who live in Ashland are natural-born to Mom and Dad; my oldest brother, Bob, is adopted, and another, Todd, is a foster brother."

"So did they think they couldn't have kids and adopted first before having kids? I mean, that is a lot for nowadays and to adopt on top of it all."

Nnugggllp, I swallow hard. *This is it, the time to be upfront and completely honest.* "Actually, my grandmother had ten kids and developed Alzheimer's when some were still young children, so the youngest went to live with the oldest siblings. My parents were already married with two kids, Karen and Jay, when they invited Bob to come and live with our family."

"What about the foster brother?" she asks, and immediately I breathe out in relief that she skipped over the whole thing with my grandmother having Alzheimer's as well as my mom.

"My brother Dan became close friends with Todd through our church and he needed a place to live, so we invited him to live with us."

"Your parents were quite generous to open up their home."

Nodding politely, I step backward into a shadow as Andy steps forward. Ralph playfully nudges Andy as Andy leans down to pick up a heavy piece of wood. Sparks jump as it is thrown on the fire.

Timidly excusing myself, I scuttle into the kitchen. *She's worried about allergies? Allergies? I wish all I had were allergies. Will they ever approve of Andy and me being together if they comprehend the truth of my tainted bloodline and questionable future?*

I strain to eavesdrop on their conversation from my safe haven. *Are they grilling Andy or trying to pry information?* I hear only muffled murmurs beyond the hum of the refrigerator.

CHAPTER 52

*

Onion Days

FOUR MONTHS AGO ANDY invited me to Marin County in order for us to be together. "You write, I'll work," he said. The winter snow of Ashland has been replaced with chilly rain down here in Corte Madera.

It is half past noon and Andy is waking after working a twelve-hour shift operating a crane on the seismic retrofit of the Richmond-San Rafael Bridge. Arriving home from work in the middle of the night, he doesn't get much sleep. I have made veggie burgers with sautéed onions and mushrooms, topped with melted cheese for a yummy and nearly gourmet meal.

"Good morning," I say, kissing him and giving him a plate of food.

"Thanks for making lunch," he says, acknowledging that I don't like to cook.

We sit on the living room floor because our apartment doesn't have a table. He slides an onion off his burger to the side of his plate, and then another, before taking a bite.

Surprised, I ask, "You don't like onions?"

Without moving, he raises one eyebrow and rotates his pupils to look at me. With a subtle head shake of annoyance, he says,

"This isn't a surprise." He returns to picking off the cheesy onions that are piled on top of the mushrooms.

My breath stops as I swallow the tiny bits of food remaining in my mouth. The sweet, caramelized onion suddenly tastes bitter and the garden burger is bland and mushy. Heat rushes to my face. By his response, I've known this for awhile, but I've totally blanked it.

"You act like I should know," I say.

"It has come up numerous times."

Slowly, I remember he always orders "no onions" on his Double-Doubles at In-N-Out Burger. He has picked them out of a stir-fry and I recall other conversations and situations where he implied or outright stated that he didn't like onions.

Shit, why didn't I remember? What is going on with me? Am I not paying attention? How long have we been dating and how many meals have we eaten together, and I don't know—or is it I don't remember—that he doesn't like onions?

He continues to pick onions with his head down. Tears somersault out of my eyes and I quickly wipe them. I sip water from a pale amber glass with my wobbly hand. *If I can hide my sobs for forty-five more minutes, he will go to work.*

Sleepy and weary of the discussion, Andy asks, "Why are you crying?" He takes a quick breath and sets down his plate.

"Because I didn't remember that you don't like onions. I feel like I have Alzheimer's already," I manage to stammer. "You said it so casually, it felt harsh."

"Well, I'm not going to lie to you if that is what you want."

Like an onion being peeled, another layer of protection is pulled off me. More feelings are uncovered; embarrassment, sadness, anxious loneliness, and the terror of Alzheimer's are the fresh juices that make my eyes gush.

He continues, "If I notice something that you forget, I'm not going to hide it. That would set up an awful precedent if you have the gene. Even if it is hard, I have to be honest."

"You are right. I don't want you to lie to me," I say. I feel like I'm going to throw up. *Holy fuck, this feels awful. Do I write down on paper all of Andy's food likes and dislikes, or does that admit defeat and the inability to trust my brain? Or do I not write it down and inadvertently set myself up for failing again? Will it give my brain the opportunity to work and remember things, or will the pressure to remember stress me out? Will I take pride in the remembering, or merely get depressed if I forget? I doubt anyone without the gene guillotine even ponders these questions. It sounds like a damn "who's-on-first" comedy, but there's no laughing here, only tears.*

"I'm sorry I put onions on it," I say. I think of Mom and when she used to forget what I liked or didn't like. I don't want him to think that I don't care about him because I didn't remember. *How do people with Alzheimer's come to terms with this lack of control of their own mind and find compassion for themselves? What do they take pride in? One of the ways I show my love for Andy is remembering what is important to him and planning those things in advance into our life. How does one with Alzheimer's disease do stuff like that?*

"You don't need to apologize; it's fine." Andy doesn't seem to mind. "It's only an onion and we are still getting to know each other."

Three weeks later, I'm helping Andy get ready for work; I'm busy making sandwiches and putting Wheat Thins and trail mix in Ziploc snack bags.

"Are you going to have a smoothie?" I ask. When he works these long hours and we spend extra time lingering playfully in bed, there is barely time to make peanut butter and jelly sandwiches before he darts out the door. I wish he would take the day off of work so we could stay in bed, letting the sweat cool on our skin.

I ask again, "Are you going to have a smoothie?" wondering if I should get out the ice cubes and fruit.

"Are you going to ask me that one more time?" His crass words cut me.

Trying to lighten the situation I ask, "Ya gonna have a smoothie?" Andy doesn't laugh or even respond. He has a disapproving frown on his face as he stares at his lunch.

Fuck—I don't remember. Is this normal to be so distracted by passion? Am I showing signs of Alzheimer's disease? I need a life partner who is gentle and can be kind despite the forgetting. I feel like I'm bleeding internally from my soul. *Do I need to be more present, talk less, and listen more? Do I need to censor what I say? Obviously my thought flow is repetitive … fuck. I hate this.*

My protective shell slides neatly into place. Now I can't wait for him to leave and don't care when he comes home. I want to be alone; at least, that is what I tell myself. The truth is, I long to be held.

CHAPTER 53

Lab Rat

HOLDING THE HEAVY GRAY door open for each other, we file inside. The sterile smell of cleaning products and fresh laundry enter my nostrils, forcing the robust outdoor air out of my lungs.

CLICK. The door shuts, locking us inside. Voluntarily admitting ourselves for two days to contribute to NIH research, I'm comforted only slightly by the presence of my siblings and my feeble hope.

Peeing in a plastic container, I hear commotion and voices in my bedroom. I'm in a lockless bathroom, so I rush to yank up my black cotton yoga pants. I wash my hands, leaving the pale yellow container on the shelf.

Turning the metal knob on the door, the room goes silent. When I enter the bedroom, five pairs of eyes stare at me.

A middle-aged woman takes two steps toward me and says, "Hello."

"Hi, what is your name?" I ask.

Drawing back, she looks insulted. "Susan," she says, staring at me expectantly.

I grope for words, trying to understand what is going on. "My name is Kate."

"Yes, yes I know, we met last year."

I don't remember her at all. She continues to stare at me, expecting something, although I'm not sure what.

My mouth is suddenly dry. I bite my lower lip. This middle-aged, self-assured woman must have been a nurse of mine during my first visit to NIH after Mom died … or did she attend the Memory Ride last year along with other NIH staff? I scan my memory. Nothing there. I try to convince myself, still nothing. There are several other staff members in the room along with my intake nurse, who is on the far side near my luggage. She is focused on me as well, watching my blank face.

I realize I must be intruding in some way. I turn to leave, sneaking out from under the scrutiny of expectant eyes.

Upon entering the hallway, another nurse walks toward me. "So you met Susan, I assume?"

"Uh, yeah," I answer hesitantly, rubbing my chin.

She smiles knowingly.

Examining her face, I realize I may have been snowballed. I timidly ask, "Is Susan my roommate?"

Continuing down the hall, she calls over her shoulder, "Yes."

I allow my body to fall back to rest on the wall, arms hanging limp. The right corner of my mouth takes a quick upswing, and I begin chuckling to myself. *Susan is the one with Alzheimer's symptoms and she tricked me into thinking that I'm the one with Alzheimer's by her well-established coping systems!*

Inside the room, I hear someone ask, "How old are you?"

Susan responds, "Why keep track anymore?"

*

Walking through the door of occupational therapy on the sixth floor, a woman with curled brown hair stands up from a round table to greet me. "Hello, you must be Kate." She looks at her watch and asks, "You are part of the Noonan family?"

"Yes, you probably worked with my mom before she died," I volunteer, trying to allow conversation so I will relax before I take the life skills test.

"Oh, I'm merely filling in for the usual person who is on vacation. But I met with one of your aunts." She glances down at a file. "Your mom had Alzheimer's disease?"

"Yes," I respond, wondering why she is even addressing this. None of the other testers asked these questions.

"Have you already found out your genetic status or are you going to find out?"

I cringe. "It is a difficult situation." I look around the room. It reminds me of a home economics kitchen with the standard appliances and an unremarkable round table. Across the room is an iron and ironing board near a washer and dryer. "I'm supposed to make a meal?"

Ignoring my question, she goes on. "I think I would want to know, but when I stop to think about it, I don't know anymore."

She is too nosy and unprofessional. I again attempt to end the conversation. "What do I have to do to complete this test?"

She looks slighted, but defers. "Make two meals that you usually make at home, such as a breakfast with eggs and coffee."

"I'm mostly vegan," I say, "so I usually eat almond butter toast with flax oil, and I don't drink coffee. I don't usually cook. I eat a lot of sandwiches." Her left eyebrow raises and her index finger taps her lips.

After agreeing on two meals, I proceed to make toast with

hot cocoa. I forget to put jam on the toast, and spill the hot cocoa while stirring it. The tester is observing me and taking notes.

Next, I make a grilled cheese sandwich, but the butter is cold. After microwaving it for twenty seconds, nothing happens, so I microwave it for forty seconds. It completely melts. As I take the plate out, butter spills off the plate and onto the floor. *Are they trying to see how many times I flub up, or is it how I move about the kitchen?*

Placing the grilled cheese on a plate, I cut it in half. Then, I pour a glass of caffeine-free Diet Pepsi in honor of Mom. Setting both on the table, I look at the tester. She is watching my every move.

"Are you finished?" she asks.

"I have to do the dishes, but that's about it. What should I do with this food?"

"Don't worry about cleaning up, that is my job. You may eat the food or leave it right there and put the other dishes in the sink."

I quickly place everything in the sink and wipe the counter and stove. "I'm not hungry. So that's it? I'm done?" I ask.

Looking at her watch she says, "Yes, I promised to get you out by three p.m. so you can meet with your *uhmm*," she clears her throat, "your genetic counselor." She raises her eyebrow, looking cleverly at me.

My jaw ripples with fury. *She fucking knew I was going to meet with a genetic counselor when I first came in and she was trying to tease information out of me.*

I glare at her, turn on my heel, and race toward the locked unit. Taking the stairs two at a time, I know if I hurry I will be able to catch Dan and warn him about her rude and prying manner. He's scheduled to meet with her immediately after me.

✳

Lying still is all that is required for the spinal tap—the easiest, but inherently the most risky test. Hating anything medically invasive, being health conscious, and believing in natural remedies, I trade off some of my values for a deeper moral obligation. Dabbing on essential oils I pray for safety, the doctor's steady hand, and a cure. As I hear the doctor walking into the room, I quickly hide away the glass bottles containing essential oils. Glass bottles are banned. They want me to store my oils behind the nurse's counter along with my vitamins, hair dryer, and nail clippers.

I feel a prick in my spine, a tiny bee sting. I'm in the fetal position, lying on my right side. Karen is sitting as close as she can without being on the bed with me. I want her closer, but the doctor is afraid of extra movement with two of us on one bed.

Slowly, a sensation like a gust of hot air moves up my spine. Although the spinal tap is intense, it's the one necessary test. The doctors say the rest of the research (blood samples, MRI, and cognitive testing) isn't worth much without the spinal tap because they are studying to find indicators of Alzheimer's disease years before symptoms are apparent. My pulse rate soars and I feel hot in my core and cold in my hands and feet.

The feeling has traveled the length of my spine and begins seeping up into the nape of my neck, until the sensation of a reverse waterfall reaches the crown of my head, sucking fluid from my forehead. Wicked pressure and a headache follow. The test is over. Tears fall onto my pillow, relief combined with pain. Karen's soft voice continues to soothe me. The doctor leaves with my gift of clear essence in little vials. My siblings are next. I lie still, thankful to be alive and participating in this research. It is one thing to know my mom had the gene and had Alzheimer's, and quite another to be face to face with my own fate right there in the Alzheimer's unit at NIH.

✳

I'm sitting, staring at the screen of an old, large, beige boxy computer that is in the corner of a tiny room. My testing monitor behind me is reading a girly fashion magazine. She gets up occasionally to measure thirty inches between my face and the screen.

This test determines eye and hand response time. An X flashes on the screen, and then a black dot followed by a red dot, and I'm to push the right button if they appear in the same place, or a left button if they appear at different locations on the screen.

Throbbing lower back pain from the lumbar puncture seems to pulse in sync with the monitor. The screen, feeble in its old age, doesn't hold a steady glow—it fades, dips, sways, surges, screams, and ever changes before my pupils as I try to simply watch the X and the red and black dots.

Once in awhile between the dots and the next X, I see the word "correct" on the screen. However, I'm sure some of the ones that are not labeled as correct are actually correct. *Is this test less about response and more about how you deal with the stress of the testing, calling things incorrect that were actually correct?*

It takes immense concentration for me to see if the dots are in the same location, and then to actually push the different buttons with my intended response. Sometimes I know they are not in the same location and in an effort to be quick, I push a button in haste, only to realize it is the wrong button.

When I don't see the word "correct," I try to recreate the memory to see if, indeed, the two dots were in the same location and I simply thought they were a few centimeters off, or if I simply pushed the wrong button.

My eyes cross and I clench them closed between the final red dot and the next X to try and see straight again. Eventually, I let them stay crossed and think maybe it will help my score to use a different part of my brain.

I have been staring at the computer for an hour, clicking right and left, when, trying through my strained vision to adjust my focus on the next X, I notice my reflection in the monitor and everything behind me. It's a new perspective. I get the next one wrong—too slow of a response.

The X that I'm supposed to be chasing with my eyes rests on my mirrored image, dead center on my forehead. It's a bit freaky. Then, a black dot and red dot appear in the same spot, as if I were Hindu. A big X is on my forehead, as if it's a sign that my brain will be deleted or X-ed out. I shudder and squint, trying to ignore the third dimension while pressing the correct button.

When I finish the sixth segment of the two-hour test, I'm asked to return to the Alzheimer's unit. I'm exhausted mentally and physically. I want to run away—or rather, walk away. The lumbar puncture has left me too sore to do much more than hobble. Yet, I'm in solidarity with my siblings, and like an old Western movie, I can't desert my blood; we are in this together.

A primal part of me pushes the buzzer outside the heavy gray door. Like a doorbell, the buzzer alerts the nurses to unlock the door, readmitting me to the Alzheimer's unit.

CHAPTER 54

Fiber Splinters

"HI, YOU MUST BE Kate. Feel free to just call me Jack," the genetic counselor says as he gets up from his chair. He has a trimmed beard and brown hair.

"Yes, hi, Jack. It's nice to meet you. Thanks for being willing to see me." I sit halfway down in the chair opposite him at the table. "Before we get started, I know one of my siblings wants to see you—they're having a tough time, but they don't have an appointment. I'm wondering if we can split the time, so we can both see you."

"That's not a problem. I should have some time tomorrow," he says, flipping open his appointment book. "I've left a wide opening for an appointment that probably won't take the whole time. What's going on?"

"The sibling's significant other is insisting that they find out their genetic status. They've had a lot of problems with their relationship and are actually taking time apart right now. During the rest of their relationship, the significant other said they didn't want to know, but now in the last couple of months, the significant other has to know in order to stay together."

Nodding while writing a note, he says, "Tomorrow, I'll call

the nurse's desk and leave a message for your sibling about what time I'm able to meet."

"Ah, that sounds good. Thanks." I have been sitting with my right foot underneath me. I move it out to settle fully into the chair.

"You obviously care a lot about your family to offer your sibling your counseling spot."

"Yeah. I hate to see them in so much pain."

"So, Kate, how about you?"

"I'm not ready to find out my status now because I'm in the process of writing a book about Alzheimer's disease and how the gene has affected me. I need to finish the book without finding out."

"I'm impressed you are writing about it. It will be quite useful to a wide audience, from Alzheimer's caregivers to professionals." Jack's words encourage me. He adds, "I wonder at the same time if your focus is too much on Alzheimer's disease and is adding stress to your life?"

I respond, "That's interesting to think about. It does increase my emotions by bringing Alzheimer's so fresh and present, but it also is healing as I'm writing and processing everything."

I continue, "I want to be sure that if I find out, my status will be completely confidential. I also want to know if NIH is utilizing one's learned genetic predisposition as a component of their testing process. For example, knowing someone's real genetic status and then telling them something different to test the power of the mind. To see if one believes they have it or don't have it, and if it will manifest or disappear accordingly." I begin to feel uneasy, because I sound paranoid. I also usually let other people talk more and I notice how proactive I'm being in this session.

"Oh, no, we could never do that. That would violate every ethical and moral standard that we are based on. Your status is completely confidential, except for the people that you choose to tell. If the doctor is concerned about some aspect of your life or if you begin to develop symptoms, the doctor will discuss that directly with you."

"I figured that's the case, but I want to be completely sure." I sit back in my chair, silent for a few moments.

"How has having the gene in your family affected you?" He doesn't look like a counselor. He appears to have a strong body, as if he does physical labor. His fingers are thick, yet smooth.

"Phew, it affects every aspect. I don't have as much confidence as I used to have. I'm not pursuing a full-time job, I don't have health insurance, but I have life- and long-term-care insurance. I have no interest in getting married or having children. I'm not saving for retirement and see little hope for my future. I live day by day."

I pause, wondering if I'm saying too much and if he is ready to lock me away, diagnosing me with severe depression.

"I'm haunted every day by symptoms or what I perceive to be possible symptoms. I'm a perfectionist and anything less could be a sign of Alzheimer's, including forgetting an errand, a name, or something at the grocery store. I keep lists of everything and put items like keys, a phone, or shoes in the same place every time I'm finished using them. I'm also hyper-vigilant of my mood, often wondering if my emotions are in a normal range given my circumstances." There is a slight tremor in my voice as I share this with him.

Jack leans forward, his head bobbing slowly forward and back. The words continue to stream out of my mouth.

"My mind is constantly analyzing in the midst of conversations. I wonder what people contemplate and how they physically move in relation to each other and who is emotionally open or closed. I see all sides of the non-spoken conversation. The down-side is it takes me longer to form my own words, and if I forget my train of thought, I worry that people see Alzheimer's symptoms in me. I get so wrapped up in Alzheimer's disease that I can't even return to the original ideas being discussed."

Jack clears his throat and asks, "Have you considered adding more to your life? Take more risks to increase your confidence level and increase your courage by taking more chances?"

"In my mind, failure of any sort is directly related to Alzheimer's. Why would I take a chance doing anything that I might fail at? It seems easier on my psyche to do things I know how to do."

Twenty minutes later, I look around the room. The intensity of the bright summer sun is subtly shifting into the late afternoon sky. My butt aches from the hard wooden chair.

"Is Andy prepared for how it may impact him if you find out your genetic status? Does he have any experience with Alzheimer's disease?"

"No. He knows a lot about my life, but he has never seen it firsthand. I have told him I might freak out and run away if I have the gene. I hate dragging him into all of this and feel that I should push him away."

"Does Andy regret your relationship?"

"He is very happy and says he wants to be with me either way."

"Repeat that again, only louder," Jack says with a faint glimmer of a smile.

"Ughh." I repeat, "No, he is very happy and says he ... umm ... wants to be with me either way." I say it louder, but my voice shakes. *Jack is definitely a counselor—making me repeat something.*

"All relationships will change with new knowledge. What is

holding you back might not be the fear of Alzheimer's, but may be the fear of the change. Who do you have to support you?"

"Besides Andy, I have my siblings; they are dealing with the same issue. However, sometimes I feel uncomfortable bringing up my fears to them as I don't want to activate their own. I also have a few close friends in whom I confide. I don't talk to many people about the entire situation."

"It would be good for you to reach out and find more friends. Let others into your life. Learn to accept support."

"I feel like a burden. The issues I deal with, most people can't even relate to. It seems better to keep it to myself. Most people know a bit about my life, but don't know the daily impact and how much it constantly affects me. If I tell someone my history, I rarely follow up and tell them how often I think about Alzheimer's disease or how it affects my every decision. In addition, finding out one's status is the hardest part, and that is of the highest level of confidentiality."

"Letting people support you gives them something also. Life is short, as you well know. You need to find a way to enjoy each day. Enjoy Andy more, engage in life more. Give and take all that life is offering you."

Jack continues, "Since you are not finding out your status right now, I suggest you focus on what you want your life to be like, and then every day take steps to get there. Get a clear picture and focus on it."

I look down at the white tissue in my hand and begin to rip accordion-like holes along the grain of the tissue. I watch the fragile fibers splinter and extend. The section damp from teardrops silently separates.

Jack says, "Imagine you are looking at a huge mural, and painted on it is your future."

I look at him, puzzled. "My future?"

He says, "What do you see down the road? What happens when you view your life—can you see where it is going?"

Unnerved, I awkwardly scoot in my chair and glance up again into his observant face. I take an uneasy breath, feeling my heart's nervous thump. Tuning in, I listen deep within myself. I can see part of the picture as I walk down the hall in my mind's eye. I report to him, "I can see the colors and movement. As I continue to look the colors meld together and the picture is no longer distinguishable; it is turning to gray. As far as I see, a dark cloud hovers over the picture, and nothing is discernable."

Tears have formed in my eyes as I hear my own voice and the eerie statement I have given. I take a tissue from the box that is conveniently located next to me on the otherwise empty table. Then, shutting down the emotion, I report matter-of-factly, "I don't really see a future. I don't see myself in it."

CHAPTER 55

Boreal

SNOW FALLS LIGHTLY AND the crisp air on my body awakens every pore. I miss the slopes of Mount Ashland since I moved to Marin County, so Andy and I are spending the day snowboarding at the Boreal Mountain Resort near Tahoe.

Andy travels on the toe edge of his board, transecting the mountain's face. Then, he switches to heel edge, moving back and forth. He is upright with his legs stiff—intentional and focused. I want to rip down the mountain cutting S's around people and over snow mounds, with my dancing hips guiding my board. Instead, I stop to wait for him, in case he falls or wants advice. I tone down my drive for speed and feel gratitude that he is accepting falling, sore muscles, and the learning process.

At the end of the day, our vehicle is one of the last remaining in the parking lot, despite the lights and availability for night skiing. Our trek home is filled with easy conversation and comments about the beauty from Boreal to Sacramento. The misty snow is opening up to stars flickering off and on, like a firefly mating ritual. Andy's round face glows alien-green in the light from the dash and I find him as handsome as ever. My heart pounds in my chest as if newly in love.

Driving over the water along Highway 37, Andy asks, "Why do all of your siblings seem to be against religion after growing up as preacher's kids?"

Surprised by his question, I stutter, "Well, I can only talk from my perception, as I haven't directly asked them this question. I think all of us believe in God or a higher power of some sort, but institutionalized religion doesn't fit for us. It was riddled with rules and expectations that we followed to the letter of the law, especially being preacher's kids. Required to set a good example, we avoided all suspicion of sin. As a fifth grader, I was not allowed to wear jeans that had a V-yoke, as it 'drew attention to my vagina' and might cause someone to backslide. We lived in constant fear that an angry, judgmental God was going to smite us down if we didn't follow His ways. After a while, our spirits grew weary of the impossible task to be perfect. Each of us gradually grew away from it in our own way and time."

"All of you seem to be angry at God for taking your father so soon," Andy observes.

"That is true. I think we all feel cheated since Dad died. If God has any compassion, why would God allow not only Mom to lose her mind, but allow us to lose Dad in the throes of it all? We had resigned ourselves to the demise of Mom, but in the battle we hadn't calculated Dad in the death toll."

A minute goes by before Andy says, "My relationship with God is the reason I'm who I am today. All the good qualities that you like about me I don't think would be part of me if it wasn't for God." An uncomfortable twinge moves inside of me as I fear a religious conversion talk—a talk I had given many times in my life, trying to save those I loved.

He continues, "That is also why I'm able to be with you today with all the uncertainty in our future surrounding Alzheimer's."

Does he worry about my spirituality and its ability to get me through hard times? It's probably true; his connection to Christianity has been influential. Often, I'm depressed or overwhelmed and Andy isn't worried at all about the future. Putting my heels up on the dashboard, the heater warms them and I press my toes onto the cool windshield.

Andy says, as if answering my unspoken question, "I'm not saying this to try and get you to change your life, but I feel like I have to acknowledge that part of me."

Quietness settles over his words while the *Gedda, Gedda, Gedda* of the diesel engine rumbles underneath the floorboards. Hundreds of red taillights curve over the next incline. Traffic is thick with powder hounds returning to the city.

Minutes later, he says, "I don't think we would be in this situation if it weren't for the Alzheimer's gene." His fingers reach out to hold my hand across the middle seat's console. I welcome his touch with an open palm caress, savoring the moment our fingers settle together.

"Why is that?"

"Well for starters, you might have married Jim."

"Yeah, maybe."

"And I know I wouldn't be living with you."

"Why is that? What's the difference?"

"I always swore I would never live with anyone before marriage, but I love you so much that I don't want to mess anything up. I want to do the best possible thing for the health and longevity of our relationship. Given the circumstances, this feels right."

"Why would you want to be with me given the possible looming pain in the future?"

Andy says, "I don't know the future, and accept that we may not retire together or spend our days traveling about. I'm not worried about it."

Feeling he doesn't get the full implication of the disease, I implore, "Andy, you have no idea what it will be like if I become angry and mean and don't realize what I'm doing."

Andy insists, "I don't know all the details of Alzheimer's, but I'm well aware that when we are fifty, you may be hugging me one minute and hitting me the next."

A wind sharper and colder than I have felt all day cuts my breath inside the heated Dodge cab as his words pierce the distance between us. Fingers of emotion grab at my throat, terror rising. Groping for words, I have none. He is more accurate than I ever wanted him to be. There was some luxury in the space of his naiveté, but now, his simple statement leaves the reality of our possible future raw, jagged, and all too revealing.

My hand stiffens and I withdraw from his touch. My heart surrenders to the intense, unexpected blow of painful, bitter truth. We finish the rest of the trip in silence.

✳

CHAPTER 56

You Look Like Your Mom

AS I ROUND THE corner into our wood-paneled living room in Corte Madera, I see my cousin Jessica, who is visiting while on a road trip during her college spring break. She is sitting on the bark-brown love seat. As I enter, her conversation with her friend, who is sitting on the couch, ceases. I stutter-step, thinking I have interrupted, but she is looking intently at me. Wonder fills her face—her mouth drops slightly, as if seeing something for the first time.

She exclaims, "Katie, you look like your mom."

Uncontrollably, I shudder as three lightning bolts strike me.

My mind jumps to the genetic links and the fear that I will end up like Mom did. I have a sudden memory of her drugged and hunched over, drooling and half asleep over a tray of food. Mom's hair is nappy and dirty and she has food on her face and pink medicine stuck in her teeth.

With the next bolt, I shiver with Mom's anger and hear her yell, "That's bullshit." Her fist is clenched in defiance.

The final memory is a zap from November 23, three years ago. Dried, tight tear lines crack on my face. I'm exhausted, lying limp next to Mom on her hospice bed, cradling her still-warm dead body.

It's an instant after Jessica spoke and I'm only three steps into the living room. Jess sees my shudder and quickly asks, "Is that bad, to look like your mom?" Then she adds, "I mean when she was young, of course." Her wide blue eyes wait for an answer, trying to be sure I'm not insulted. Her hair, a silky chestnut-brown with a reddish hue, is the same length as mine, and skims her lower shoulder blades. She is biting her fingernails.

I cringe, knowing she is proud of Fran, her recently deceased mom, and that she wants to be like her—a smart, powerful, outspoken, devout Christian. Her mom and my mom were the first of their generation to get Alzheimer's disease. I don't want to influence Jess with my anti-Alzheimer's obsession, so I stammer, "Uh, no I guess not."

I continue into the kitchen. Once out of her sight, I grab the edge of the old wood cabinets with copper handles to steady myself, and close my eyes. *How did I let my true feelings show?* Chatter starts again in the living room. It is deafened by the blood pulsating in my ear drums and the words—*You look like your mom. You Look Like Your Mom. YOU LOOK LIKE YOUR MOM!* reverberating inside my skull.

CHAPTER 57

Everyday Life

PLAYING AS A FORWARD, I chase the ball into the other team's penalty box at the Marin Women's Soccer League tournament. Weightless, I run, half floating, as sweat trickles out of my pores. The other team's center midfielder has passed it backwards to the fullback, and I follow to try and steal the ball or force a weak play. The powerful defendant nails the soccer ball; it would have traveled half the length of the field if it didn't hit my noggin ten feet from her. *Bam.* The blast squarely smacks the side of my skull, knocking my teeth together and sending me to the ground in a solid *thud* while the ball returns like a rocket to the defendant.

Tweet. The ref stops the game, seeing me fall in a heap. I crawl, shaking my head, and claw the soft spring dirt and tufts of grass. Regaining my vision, I push my teetering body up to stand. I wobble-jog to the edge of the field amid other players yelling "Stay down," and "Are you okay?" In the background I hear a whisper, "Yeowch, that was a doozy."

At the sideline, where we have two subs, I insist that I'm fine and ask for my water bottle. If I take a break now, I will obsess over Alzheimer's. Guzzling the cool liquid, I'm aware how dangerous soccer can be, and possibly more so for me than the other players on this field. I have heard that heading the ball and any other head trauma is detrimental to people predisposed to Alzheimer's disease. Unless I am within goal-scoring range, I avoid headers of my own volition. But inevitably, by being on the field, I still take whoppers. Replacing the black lid on my blue Nalgene, I toss it into my evergreen bag beyond the white chalk line.

Turning to resume the game, I wonder if the sheer exhilaration of playing is worth the impact in the long run. Something comes alive in me when I play soccer. The sensation of ecstasy vibrates through my bones in ways that I feel only in the rare instances when my physical body is totally engrossed. This allows my mental hamster wheel to shut down, loosening the heavy burden. Shaking my throbbing skull one more time, I attempt to stop the seepage of Alzheimer's thoughts and hope my meditative zone will return once again.

Eliza, my high school friend, is visiting before Andy and I move to Astoria, Oregon. With dark blonde hair and speckled blue eyes, she is articulate, introspective, and quick to laugh. We are sitting on the couch after dinner and I'm playing with my hair, looking at the split ends that have accumulated since my last haircut more than eight months ago.

I say, "Some strands of my hair are black, and I have only begun to notice it in the past couple of years."

Eliza exclaims, "I have that, too."

I separate out a thin, pale blonde hair and a thick, jet-black hair to show her the intense difference. "It's hard to believe they grow on the same scalp."

"I know what you mean. I always pluck the black ones."

"I have thought of pulling them out, but I keep mine. I like having them there. I'd prefer perfect blonde hair, but having black hair gives me hope that maybe I share more genes with Dad than I do with Mom."

✳

CHAPTER 58

Held Up by Piling

AFTER DROPPING OFF THE U-Haul trailer in Warrenton, Oregon, we are relieved of the last burdensome aspect of our recent move to Andy's hometown. We are at a restaurant famous for its fish and chips and nearly any seafood that is fried. Located on the Columbia River, the restaurant is held up by piling. An old boiler stands two hundred feet offshore, historically marking the cannery that used to operate at this site.

The patrons are wearing Carhartt clothing, and some are very overweight. People here are tough—a blue-collar community, proud and hard working. The floor shakes beneath the petite hostess as she greets customers and marches them to their tables.

Our food arrives, towering over the white plates. Delicately, I pry apart a piece of the golden battered fish, and steam billows out of the center.

"Careful, it is hot and takes a while to cool," Andy cautions.

"Yeah, I can see that. I'm blowing on it to refrigerat—" I stop mid sentence. My body stiffens.

"What did you say?" He leans closer to listen.

Tears spring from my eyes as I look at his body crouched near me. It's the words, mixed up and misplaced, that terrify me.

The ones I usually catch and transform before they fall out of my mouth.

"I said, I wwas blowing on it t-to re-refri …" He nods and I don't have to finish.

"I thought I was the only one to say stuff like that," he says playfully.

A cool, wet trickle continues down my face, even though I have dammed it up with my napkin. "That has been happening a lot in the past couple of days, and it scares me. It's one of the signs."

"Yeah, the difference is I think I'm a dumb-ass whenever I do something like that, but you … it means something to you."

CHAPTER 59

Full-Blown Panic

ELIZA IS VISITING FOR a few days and we are stretching on the tan-peppered carpet in the living room of Andy's float house on Blind Slough. Our tight, sleepy muscles lack exercise due in part to the rainy weekend's continual downpour.

Eliza is serene. Lost in thought, she twists her puckered lips to the edge of her cheek and says, "You called me within hours after my mom died. I was surprised you found out so quickly. First, that your dad knew, and then that he was able to contact you when you were living at Kripalu." She moves into the pigeon yoga stretch. "I was in the middle of calling relatives."

Eliza's mom died a couple years after Eliza graduated high school. We used to take walks and talk about our moms' illnesses, hers with cancer, mine with Alzheimer's. When Dad called Kripalu Yoga Center, he must have said it was an emergency because someone found me while Dad waited. After talking with Dad, I immediately called Eliza.

"You seemed so collected. When I asked if you wanted me to come to the funeral, you said no, you had lots of people around and wouldn't get much time with me anyway." I'm resting flat on my stomach with my head turned toward Eliza, my hand cushioning my face.

"I was collected?" Eliza asks, her low eyebrows wrinkling. "I don't remember that at all. Everything's a blur."

We are silent for a moment. She switches legs and goes into pigeon pose again, her face descending toward the floor as the pink rims of her eyelids redden and begin watering. She picks at the flecked carpet fibers with alternating hands. Whispering, she says, "I wish I had asked you to be at my mom's funeral."

"Me too," I say, nodding. I hold her gaze, taking a lung-stretching breath. My voice delicately whispers, "Now I see how important that was. It was a pivotal moment in your life and we talk about death and dying on a regular basis. I wish I could have witnessed the funeral in support of you then as well as now."

Wo woo—wooo Wooooo. The shiny black tea kettle on the stove emits stuttered whistles.

"The water is ready, but I don't want to lose the tone of this conversation," I say, acknowledging her palpable tears as we both scramble into the kitchen.

Gushing white steam, the kettle is shrieking. Turning off the burner, I lift the spout cover to fill our waiting mugs with boiling water.

The equilibrium of the house changes with a nearly imperceptible sway from the wake of an invisible passing skiff in the black night. The zoom of the motor fades as it travels down the slough towards the Columbia River. The bright wood cabinets glow yellow from the in-set ceiling light, and our reflection is navy in the clear glass windows that have darkened since the sun dropped below the horizon.

"Is there more on your mind that you want to talk about?" I inquire as I dunk our tea bags.

"I'm still surprised how inadequate I feel at supporting others in the death process, even after going through it myself," Eliza says. "For example, I'd call my friend Ryan when his mother was dying and leave a message. Then, I waited for a return call before calling again. But when I was in the depths of everything with my mother, I had no energy to return calls."

"I don't think you can beat yourself up over that. In some ways it's common courtesy. It's also the responsibility of those grieving to communicate their wishes. When your mom was sick, you told me specifically that you didn't have the energy to call, but you liked talking to me when I called you."

"I understand what you're saying, but I feel like I should've been more available. Kate, I still don't know what to say at funerals."

"Sometimes it's best to not say anything at all. Remember all the awful things people said to us in the funeral line, like 'Cheer up' and 'At least you have a strong family'? What did they say to you?"

"One guy walked up to my dad and said 'It only gets worse from here.'" Eliza imitates the man with scrunched eyebrows and a vigorous, stern headshake. Then, batting flirty eyes she continues, "My aunt's friend, who was sort of forced through the funeral line, said with surprise, 'There are lots of good-looking people here. Are they all from the North Country?'" We both chuckle, then Eliza says, "The best thing to do if you don't know what to say is to keep your mouth shut. Give a hug or move on."

"I haven't been faced with wondering what to say at memorial services," I say, thinking about the past two years. Then, I realize the absurdity of that statement, remembering my Aunt Kathi's death was the same day as Mom's, and I add, "Well, I guess I had Mom and Fran's funerals."

Fran? Wait—she didn't die the same day as Mom; it was Kathi, my other aunt. Mom and Kathi died nine hours apart. I'm used to saying the names Mom and Fran together, as they were the first two of their generation diagnosed with Alzheimer's disease. *Fran's still alive. I screwed up my words.* In less than a minute, I've shattered into a severely confused state fueled by Alzheimer's panic.

I re-state, "I mean Mom and Kathi's funeral."

Wait … Fran was in a care facility when Mom died, but she is *dead now.* I'm locked in overdrive, trying to figure out why my brain is not working right. Why can't I remember which aunt is dead? Is this malfunction another sign of Alzheimer's disease? *I'VE GOT TO PULL MYSELF TOGETHER.* When I speak, I'm usually much more careful and calculated; with Eliza, I have let down my guard.

Sheer panic seizes me as I ask aloud from the downward-spiraling mental merry-go-round, "Did I go to Fran's funeral?" White sweat sears my skin. Eliza's face elongates as her jaw drops inside her closed lips. *I know I should know this. Okay, quit talking out loud, I'm saying too much.*

"I'm having a total panic attack," I confide as I blink uncontrollably, my vision darting in all directions, searching for internal answers. She is watching me as my mind spews out garbage like a computer gone haywire, indiscernible symbols scrambling the screen as emotions kamikaze my thought process. *Yes! I was there; I remember what I wore and spending time with my cousins Phil and Jess, who were in their early 20s. THIS IS A SIGN OF ALZHEIMER'S DISEASE. YOU FUCKED UP YOUR WORDS. THEN, IT TOOK A FULL SECOND TO REMEMBER WHEN FRAN'S FUNERAL WAS AND THAT YOU ATTENDED IT. THAT IS NOT SOMETHING YOU SHOULD FORGET.*

Eliza is gawking at me, waiting for me to finish talking. *What was I talking about? Quit thinking about Alzheimer's and focus on the issue at hand. Yes, okay, it was about Fran's funeral.*

"Yeah, I went to Fran's funeral," I say, finally breaking the silence. I'm not sure who is more relieved, Eliza or me. "When I arrived in Pennsylvania, I met up with my sister Karen. We brought Jess and Phil Oreo ice cream and UTZ sour cream and onion chips—both items, I remember, Fran always kept on hand. We also brought a box of Puffs, as tissues rapidly vanish during times of mourning and sandpaper generic brands make noses raw."

Eliza and I look at each other again. I force myself to hold eye contact, although I feel a smidge shifty, like I'm trying to sneak under the radar screen that's flashing a bold red warning light over my head.

"That sounds like a great way to be supportive of your cousins. But getting back to the panic attack, I forget some things like that as well," she says with sincerity.

I look away, closing my eyes. Nothing anyone says can tame this fear-based boa constrictor that is eating me alive.

Still feeling the need to prove myself, I continue, "It was the night before Fran's funeral and Jess was sick of interacting with so many people. Everyone was asking how she was doing and she wanted to respond, 'My mom died, how do you think I'm doing?' She already had people saying the wrong things to her and she wanted to tell everyone, 'Don't say anything; just bring chocolates.'"

"Phil, on the other hand, said everyone expected him to be sad and depressed about losing his mother, but mostly he was relieved it was over, and to him, Fran had been gone for a long time. He couldn't visit her because she didn't recognize him as her own grown son. Instead, to Fran, he resembled a relative who abused her when she was a young child and therefore, Phil's presence instigated fear and anger. Intense, huh?"

Eliza nods and doesn't say anything.

CHAPTER 60

Tormented Dreams

FOUR YEARS HAVE PASSED since Mom's death; my life is nearly paralyzed by the fear of Alzheimer's disease. Taunting me, Alzheimer's looms on the horizon, threatening to strike, out of reach, but always within sight. My writing seems to be triggering nightmarish dreams.

It is my second night visiting Eliza in New York City. We are having our own private writing vacation to inspire and bounce ideas off each other. I love seeing Eliza, but don't love NYC. The last time I visited was immediately following the family genetic study at NIH, where I had the lumbar puncture. My body hurt and I walked so slowly that the whole city seemed to leave me in the dust. The good parts were eating a chewy gyro and smelling subway exhaust with a migraine. This time, I want to remember the city in a different light. I force myself to go out for walks to get to know her Brooklyn neighborhood and release the long hours of writing about Alzheimer's disease. Despite my efforts, tension builds anyway and creeps out in my dreams.

In my dream, wind blows against the youthful but emotionally tattered countenance of a young woman; her hair swirls in all directions before smacking her face. The rain-drenched trench coat hangs heavy on her small frame. Lowering her head with brows wrinkled, she shelters a swaddled baby. The baby's nose and cheeks are red and it cries out, "*Waaah, Wah, WAAaaaahh.*" The mother warmly kisses the cold cheeks.

Nearby on the narrow jetty, an old woman trips but doesn't fall. The young mother yells, "Come now, Grandma, we must get inside." The waves are crashing at the far end of the rocks and the downpour is driven diagonal by the blustery weather. The older woman vacantly looks at the young mother without recognition before staring at the sky while the rain pelts her wrinkled skin. She stumbles backward. Catching her balance, she turns towards the storm and ocean, spreading her arms wide. The breeze catches her garment and slinks in through the buttons and up underneath. Billowing like a kite, her sleeves and coat slap violently in the wind storm. Her body begins to shake as the next gust nearly knocks her off her feet. Rotating away from the wind, she hunkers down in a squat, taking shelter behind a jetty boulder.

The young mother returns again and grasps the old feeble hand. "Come, Grandma, come with me. I can't carry you. Please come. Please."

The elderly lady stays seated on her haunches, rocking and muttering to herself. Facing into the wind, the baby begins to scream through a wide mouth that covers most of her scrunched red face. "*AAAAHHHHHHHaaa, ahhhh.*" Her hat is pulled down to her invisible eyebrows and tied tight under her tiny chin.

Turning again from the gale, the young mother releases the boney, shivering hand, sheltering her baby with the brown trench coat. The old lady continues muttering nonsense. A tear falls from the young mother's cheek and plunks onto the yellow fleece baby blanket as she is forced to leave her own mother.

At the end of the jetty on the edge of the sand, the young woman turns again to the dark mound, nearly indistinguishable from the various boulders. She screams at the top of her lungs to be heard over the weather, "Mom, please come home." The blob settles further between the rocks. As another strong gust thrusts the young woman and child further away, they vanish in the turbulent night.

Waking with a shudder, I glance hastily around the room. The metallic scent of fear wafts out from under the covers. My body is sweaty. I look down at the smooth flesh on my 30-year-old hand to reassure myself it is only a dream.

Eliza and I are walking home through the chilly Brooklyn night. I pull my black dress coat taut around my body. Tonight I did my first open mic reading at a bookstore. It was a small gathering of about ten people, all strangers to me, except Eliza. I feel naked, as if I have been stripping. My voice shook, but it usually does. People either shifted uncomfortably with the intensity of my story, or they were riveted, unable to take their gaze off me. I hope, despite my excitement, I will be able to sleep tonight without the nightmares that continue to haunt me.

Three hours later, I wake, my mind replaying the dream.

I'm standing near a white, embroidered lace couch and love seat in a fancy home. I have never been in this home before, but know one of my siblings lives here.

Suddenly, I start bleeding from my arms and wrists. No one

else is in the room. I don't know what caused the bleeding—I don't have any old wounds and I didn't get cut on anything. I am gushing blood. Trying to minimize the damage, I put my arms into my clothing and maneuver my lower body underneath so it will keep the warm liquid on my body and off the couch. But the white couch is already stained. I'm distressed that I'm leaving a permanent mark. I look at the stained couch and realize that what I assumed was blood is actually ink.

Is writing so much a part of me now that ink has become my life blood? Does this dream imply that if my writing is released into the world, it will stain the lives of those around me? Do I need to continue writing because it pulses in my blood? Or do I stop because it affects others?

POSTSCRIPT

✳

I AM NO LONGER the same person who wrote this book. The courage it took to step out of hiding has opened numerous opportunities. Now, I try to say *YES!* even if I am scared. Hope is slowly returning. Not hope that I will be saved from this disease, hope that I will enjoy more moments when I run, dance, play, hug, touch, love. Hope that life can be tolerable and even enjoyable.

During the composition of this book, I was extremely concerned with every detail, that everything in my memory and my notes be impeccably recorded. After writing about the green wrought-iron garbage containers with arrowhead points in Lithia Park that I remember from ten years ago, I recently returned to the park and, to my disappointment, found there were no such trash receptacles. Instead, there are brown wooden slats embracing the removable containers. Is my memory flawed? Has there been a remodel? Do I leave out the description of the trash cans altogether, or do I fall into the memoir category of "creative non-fiction"?

There are two sides to this hypersensitivity to accuracy. First, wanting to be sure every detail is precise, I have taken time combing my journals and audio tapes. I want people to believe my experience and not doubt it by some minor detail that is incorrect. The second side to my fearful obsession with perfect memories is to ensure my brain is functioning properly. Any glimmer of faltering sends me into a deadly tailspin, threatening the vitality of this book and, in turn, my very life.

Some of Mom's abilities and conversation may seem out of place, but it is mostly in chronological order. One day, she was crystal clear and then the next, a garbled, jumbled mess. One minute she was unresponsive, then, the next, walking. That seems to be the nature of Alzheimer's. Sometimes the brain makes the connections, and other times the "wires get crossed," as Mom used to say in the early years.

Additionally, when I write about scenes in which I'm not even present, I include the individual's usual mannerisms and behaviors, yet I can't say for certain that this person bit the inside of his or her cheek at that exact moment. However, it is my best guess from the description of events and our shared experiences.

Dan was not mentioned during Mom's imminent death, which may lead the reader to believe he was uncaring or insensitive. The opposite is true; he purposefully stayed away to not disturb her process. Due to their strong connection and her miraculous healings in his presence, he thought if he showed up while she was dying, she might have opened her eyes and gotten up out of bed.

To capture the look and intensity of faces, especially my siblings, I would imitate the face I remember them making and then, with a mirror in hand at my keyboard, attempt to paint that facial expression with words. Forcing my face into the selected contortion would simultaneously raise the reciprocal emotion inside of me. Not only did I recall the experiences in my brain as I transferred the stories into my computer, but I relived the events through my emotions and body sensations.

The noises throughout the book were created from mimicking the sounds I heard on the recordings and from Mom's actual voice. I would recreate the sounds until I could find the letters that would replicate those nuances.

The intensity of both of these practices would bring me to tears over and over. I often wondered if writing wasn't healthy for me.

Refusing to read any other books while I was writing may have been a bit extreme, but I didn't want to interrupt or change my own voice. Being incredibly sensitive, I also didn't want to be intimidated by another author who has a beautifully written book when mine was still in the disjointed stage; nor did I want to read about death or Alzheimer's disease, because I wanted to be sure I included the experiences I thought were important, described in my own words.

The end result? The book is finished. I plan to schedule an appointment to find out my genetic status; however, I'm not sure I will be able to follow through. I am still terrified.

If I do manage to get my results, I doubt I will tell anyone outside of the tightest circle of support. Being uncommonly tragic, it is great gossip material. I understand that the knowledge affects the secret holders. It is so intense and disturbing that most support people need support themselves. A friend who potentially carried a genetic disease found out with much relief that she didn't carry the offending gene. Ironically, this friend faced anger and criticism from a confidant because the confidant felt that she had been lied to by being an emotional support for something that didn't exist.

Regardless of the outcome, the process of finding out is still a traumatic event. Realistically, anger will flare out toward anyone who asks about my status. It is not for public knowledge, nor should it be. Social graces are necessary in dealing with genetic diseases, as they are for AIDS.

Fran Powers, my aunt, gave a face to early-onset Alzheimer's disease in front of Congress and on many TV programs. I am giving a face to people haunted by genetic mutations. I imagine it is similar to being stalked by a serial killer. I already know his tactics; I just don't know if I can escape.

ACKNOWLEDGMENTS

Thank you:

MY FAMILY AND ESPECIALLY my siblings: for giving me your blessing to tell this story; I am grateful for your love, touch, connection, and care. I'm thankful we are still friends despite the turmoil and heartache we have endured.

My extended families: The Noonans for your outspoken, proactive public faces and courage in the wake of devastation including media attention and publicity, starting the Memory Ride, giving talks about living wills and end-of-life issues, being involved in research, and speaking to elected officials. The Preskenises for your quiet but constant support.

My loves: Andy for confidentiality, emotional support, balance, keeping me grounded, enabling me to have concentrated writing time. Jim, who played with me, loved me, spoke your truth, and tried to get me to focus on the present.

My allies: Karen, my best friend, for tea, walks, phone calls, and support beyond comprehension. Eliza, for numerous edits, shared writing retreats and my first public reading. Laura, who visits, calls, sends me cards, and continually cheers me. Jessie, who listens, tells the truth, and supports me. Margaret, for love despite time or distance. Susan, for holding me in your heart. Wyatt, my first writing partner, for being gentle. My Facebook and email friends, for your support and promoting the book.

My writing coach: Lisa Alpine, who dances with me, honored my voice, patiently edited alongside me, and assisted in the transformation of my journals and audio tapes into snapshot chapters. I wouldn't be here without your wisdom and encouragement.

My team: To my first two anonymous readers, for plunging into the depths of emotion and giving useful feedback. Lucas Balzer for friendship, website design, technical support, and photographs. Amberly Finarelli for professional edits, explanation of grammar, and allowing my voice. Jerry Ascierto for fast, professional copy and format editing. Terri Haas for interpretive logo design. Christopher Briscoe for an artistic vision in photography. Joel Friedlander for book formatting and guru-like blog updates. Joshua Tallent for answering your phone and for ebook formatting.

CNN's Felipe Barral: for choosing me to be part of your documentary, "Filling the Blank." Your belief in my book inspired me to finish and assured me it was worth telling.

Kickstarter: for accepting my project, allowing me to raise the funds needed to publish this book.

The film production company: for generously donating time and talent to create my Kickstarter video and profile shots. It's a treat I would not otherwise have been able to afford.

The Kickstarter backers: without your comments and donations, I would still be floundering. I am honored you chose to spend your hard-earned money to support this book.

101 Backers on Kickstarter:

Susan Tryon, Stephanie Day, Eryc Noonan, Joe Gecsey, Julie Lawson, Bridget E. Billings, Diana Bihoreau, Deb Pierson, Lisa Alpine, Sarah Graves Hines, Brandy Ritz, Sandra Yingling, Kevin Korobko, Joan Bartlett, Sandra Cain, Rick, Joyce Keidel, Cherise, Elaina McWilliams, Cassie and Jay Preskenis, Marisa Lyon, Jim

Quinby, Trish Smith, Amy and Dan Preskenis, Crystal Bashore, Susan Frey, Tamara Marston, Luke C. Miller, Dean Mueller, Jesse Spry, Andrew Peitsch, Ron Rezek, Marcy Henry, Carol Tierney, Danielle Hoff, E C B, Sally Callahan, Wendy Moore, Irene Hammer-McLaughlin, Melissa, Kulsum, Jolene Hurley, Michael, Kristine Cole, Julie Berry, Glenn Perrin, Kerry Ward, Sheila Noonan, Shayne Vacca, Victoria Anchipolovsky, Tara, Robb Nunn, Abolitionist, Robert and Jan Cayless, Ed Hensley, Amie Cohen, Kate Hoffmann, Courtney and Karim, Peter Burnash, Patty Barbato, Chelsie Lawson, Melissa Noonan, Brenda Irby, Kathy Ladouceur, Jeanne Burnash, katmandu56, James Turnbull, Sara, Shelly Pike, Michael Korobko, Kate Begonia, Julie, Guy and Karen, Jolynne Shannon, Ashtara Silunar, Kim Hunter, Barb Estoos, Daniel Wehking, Roxpatton, Darcy Buckley, Karla Hornstein, Jennifer Murphy, Trish, Sarah Callahan, Alvaro Fernandez, Jamie Tyrone, Pascale, Donna Perrin, Leah Farr, Jessica Hodge, Fred Windholz, Jason Fullan, Colleen Slowey, Lewis Winter, Janay Kneeland, Kristin, John Noonan, Jessie Monter, E. Carol Jefford, Brian Caruth, Damiana Thompson.

ABOUT THE AUTHOR

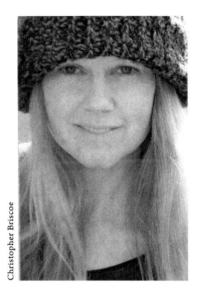

Christopher Briscoe

AFTER GRADUATING FROM ST. Lawrence University, Kate Preskenis's life took a drastic turn from pursuing social and environmental justice to mitigating the chaotic world of her mother's genetically inherited Alzheimer's disease, to ultimately grappling with her own genetic status.

Journaling since she could form sentences, Kate charted her emotions, relationships, and experiences. Imbedded in these diaries are her mother's first Alzheimer's symptoms of unexplained behavior and emotional oddities, continuing to her mother's last breath. The early death of her parents combined with the innovative capability of gene testing led Kate to value and share this unique documented history.

Residing in southern Oregon, Kate waits tables at a fine-dining restaurant. Writing, working out, going to church, dancing, and connecting with cherished family and friends keeps her body strong, spirit light, and heart open.

www.katepreskenis.com

CPSIA information can be obtained at www.ICGtesting.com
Printed in the USA
BVOW040423060612

291902BV00001B/3/P